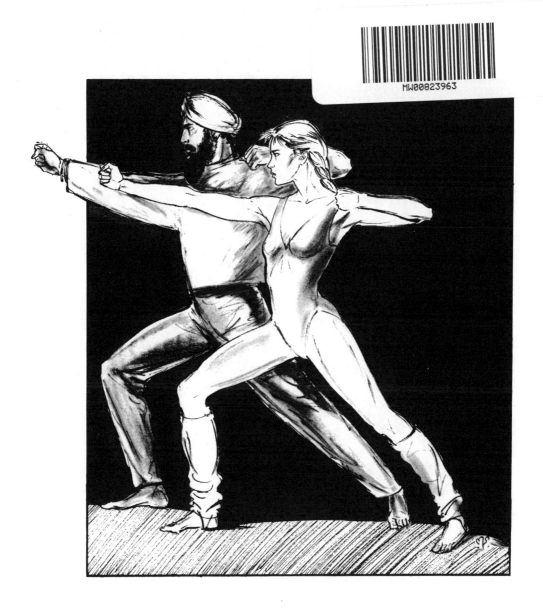

KUNDALINI YOGA
for Body, Mind, & Beyond

by Ravi Singh

KUNDALINI YOGA
for Body, Mind, & Beyond

by Ravi Singh

Published by White Lion Press
225 E. 5th St. #4D
New York, NY 10003

All illustrations to text by Marsha Silvestri (Ram Das Kaur)
Drawing opposite dedication page by Darlene Margeta
Front/Back Cover designed by Ravi Tej Singh Khalsa
Cover Model - Cara Peloso

Special Thanks to: Guru Charan Singh Khalsa, Mark Canaan, Cara Peloso, and all my
compatriots on this most noble of paths for their inspiration, example and support.

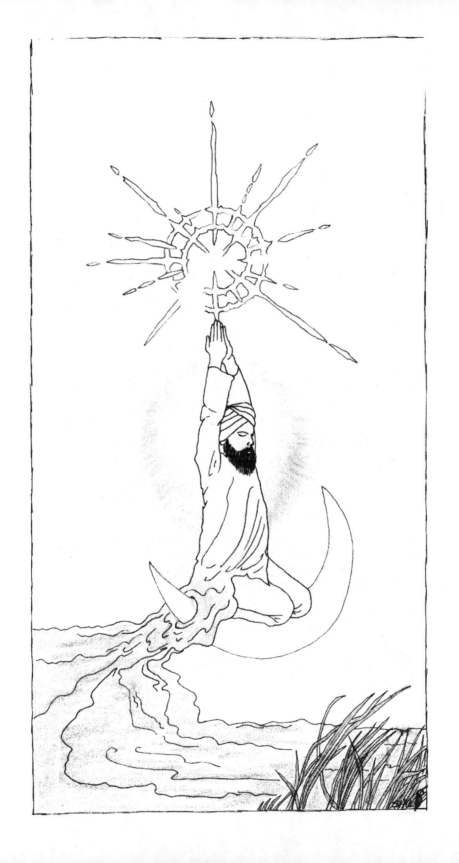

DEDICATION

To Yogi Bhajan--

A Teachers' Teacher,
A Warrior of Peace
and of Truth,
Through Whose Sacrifice
and Mastery,
This Sacred Science
Of Kundalini Yoga
Has Been Ceded
To Us--

May We,
The Beneficiaries
Of This Legacy,
In this Workshop of Time & Space,
Cherish, Preserve,
And Share
These Teachings,
With An Open Heart,
In God's Will,
And By God's Grace.

CONTENTS

Preface

Introduction   1

Chapter 1   Getting Started   6

Chapter 2   How to Use this Book   20

Chapter 3   Beginners' Sets   22

Chapter 4   O My Healthy Back   45

Chapter 5   Flexible and Free   55

Chapter 6   Navel Power   66

Chapter 7   Warrior Workout   74

Chapter 8   Digestible You   90

Chapter 9   What To Do for the Sugar Blues   97

Chapter 10   Have a Heart   101

Chapter 11   Bright and Beautiful   107

Chapter 12   Pick Me Up Exercises   113

Chapter 13   When Stress Gets the Best of You What To Do   117

Chapter 14   Best Before Bed   124

Chapter 15   Get Down to Get Up   132

Chapter 16   Diving for the Blue Pearl   139

Chapter 17   Long Live You   146

Chapter 18   Beauty from Within   151

Chapter 19   Manpower   165

Chapter 20   Beyond Sex Together   177

Chapter 21   The Inside Story   187

Appendix   204

PREFACE

by GURUCHARAN SINGH KHALSA, Ph.D

Ravi Singh has done it! He's created a practical guide book that gives you the technology and impetus to break the trance-like treadmill that living with minimum energy induces. Here is the HOW-TO Book that gives you the energy you need to fill your life with strength, success, and spirit.

These workouts are an invitation to life. They lead you to the realization that you have the resources within you to excel. This is not a collection of techniques which counsel you to withdraw from life, or limit your activity to reduce stress. It says, "Here is is the means to tap the inner energy which rests dormant in your nervous and glandular systems." With that energy, which is called "Kundalini," every challenge becomes an opportunity, every experience a resource, and every moment of life a creative endeavor.

The Kundalini Yoga Ravi Singh presents is not theoretical. It's a pragmatic daily practice which leads to the victory of your identity over the pressures of life and the impulses of your emotions. As human beings, our birthright is happiness, our destiny is success, but all too often, our choice is to fall short of our own potential. Either our concentration to hold a goal fails, under the pressure of too many distractions, the patience which comes from self-esteem and clarity is absent, or another feeling or emotion betrays our original intention.

When our energy is strong, our identity and awareness stay steady and ready to serve us. We can create and enjoy the imprint of our spirit and consciousness in everything we do and are. Yogi Bhajan, the acknowledged Master of this Yoga, has often said that the highest formula for people who wish to be happy, healthy, and fulfilled is KEEP UP!, that regardless of circumstances, there is a deeply founded security and faith that sustains you. Kundalini Yoga will give you this foundation.

The techniques which Ravi Singh has collected give you hardiness. Hardiness is an attitude of spirit which helps you to create constancy in life. With hardiness you can master the impact of stress without retreating from activity.

There are always two ways to approach life and the goals we have in life. One is the short path, which is seemingly easy. It is usually a gambler's dream which results in immediate but fleeting rewards. It gives you a vision which disappears in the light of dawn. The other way is a path that is just as accessible but longer. It is arduous, but fills you with nobility, strength, and inner realization. It uses gradual self-discipline to give you the freedom to maintain your gains.

Consider the two ways of getting to the bottom of a cliff. You can just jump and get to the bottom quickly, and beat everyone else. It's an intense experience you can shout about. You seem to have the power to fly, and you capture everyone's attention for the short time you travel. But in the end you fall to pieces. Your identity has not been maintained. You've gained nothing.

The other way is to learn rock climbing from a skilled mentor. It takes a little more time and patience. You must learn specific skills. Your original dream was to be able to get to the bottom of a cliff. You never anticipated having to learn about ropes, crapons, safety lines, muscular stamina, and group cooperation. But in the end you open yourself to the new and strange things which will help you fulfill your dream. Then you can climb down the cliff and enjoy the many new perspectives and discoveries that the measured descent gives you. You experience a sense of control and self-esteem which fills you with warmth you can share.

And there you are, at the end of your climb, not even winded, perspiring with pleasure and accomplishment, able to repeat the climb up and down as often as you want, and to teach it and explore with others, your identity and self in one piece, at peace.

It is in that tradition of the second path, growth through cultivation, that Ravi Singh has give so much to you in this book. Many of the sets are short. and energizing, but they build you up gradually into a true experience of your higher potential. They give you health, a mental attitude of flexibility and positivity, and the habit of trust in the spirit within you. They put you on the path of strength.

When you are full of your strength, your radiance and commitment ignite a similar fire in others. That fire is passed from person to person Its like lighting a great bonfire on the darkest of nights. People come out of the dark from every direction to share its warmth. Many tell stories, share knowledge, and exchange kindnesses in the light. New resources and fuel are offered to further your purpose. Many take from the fire to start new campsites Ravi Singh has taken the light from a great fire and now passes it on to you.

To Guru Ram Das and Yogi Bhajan who have preserved and passed on this knowledge, I bow with gratitude. To Ravi Singh who is a high quality Teacher of these energetic treasures I thank for keeping up and completing this book and for serving the many students he has taught and will teach To you the reader and student I share with you the anticipation of a good beginning as you master these techniques; and I look forward to your experience of self-mastery when you can elevate all with your spirit.

Gurucharan Singh Ph.D, Yogi, Psychotherapist, and Author, has fused the most profound aspects of Eastern disciplines and Western technologies. He's taught a course in called the Psychology of Yoga at M.I.T and U.C.L.A, and Kundalini Yoga and Meditation worldwide.

INTRODUCTION

All of us fantasize about what we'd like to do or be. In order to "make the fantasy real," we need some energy to work with. In the yoga tradition, this creative catalyst, or energy of your highest potential, is called Kundalini. Some have called this "spirit rising," or the motivating, evolutionary force within you.

I'm sure at times you've experienced sudden inspiration, the ability to complete complicated tasks easily, or clear insights which give your life direction and meaning. Possibly you've played a tennis match beyond your normal capacity, written a beautiful poem in a seemingly effortless way; or for no discernible reason, felt a kind of exaltation in light of which your most pressing problems look small. These are all indicative of an experience which is a legacy guaranteed to each of us.

The key word here is experience. It's been said,"If you haven't experienced something it's not true." So, it's one thing to read endless books on philosophy, self-improvement, and spirituality; in fact this may constitute an important first step. The real results though, come to those who honestly work on themselves systematically and consciously.

What Kundalini Yoga offers is a technology which can help you be the best that you can be. Many of us who've been practicing these techniques have seen that if you get everything covered, by bringing health and balance to your body, mind, and being, then you'll be covered; the Universe will underwrite your efforts. In other words, things will fall into place for you.

Kundalini Yoga is called the Yoga of Awareness. It helps you understand what you need to improve the quality of your life. Also, Kundalini Yoga supplies the energy and focus to attain and maintain these things.

The effects of Kundalini Yoga vary somewhat with each practitioner, or more accurately each person will probably be aware of certain benefits given his/her needs and expectations.

Overall though, you can expect the following through the consistent practice of Kundalini Yoga:

IMPROVED FUNCTIONING OF ALL BODILY SYSTEMS - It's not easy to make a sale when your gastritis is flaring up. Kundalini Yoga, in conjunction with the appropriate lifestyle adjustments, will put your cardio-vascular, digestive, nervous, lymphatic, glandular, and all other systems in proper working order.

STRENGTH - Muscular development is a small part of what strength really is. True strength also entails endurance, flexibility, and will. Ultimately, strength is a steady mind built on faith in your own unlimited potential.

BEAUTY - I've seen Kundalini Yoga Yoga transform many non-descript bodies into sleek physiques. Beyond this though, your beauty is your radiance and the impression you leave in the hearts of others. Kundalini Yoga is one of the only exercise systems that recognizes the importance of glandular balance in relation to physical and mental health. This has a direct bearing on your ability to look and feel great.

A CONSISTENT SENSE OF WELL BEING - This comes as a result of the increased energy and relaxation which Kundalini Yoga engenders, and from the process of self-discovery and confidence you feel when you pay attention to your inner life.

EMOTIONAL BALANCE - This attribute helps you to be master of your life and not allow subjective mental states to cloud your ability to make clear decisions and act in accordance with your true values.

HEIGHTENED SENSORY AWARENESS - The ability to touch, taste, feel, and see with sensitivity, and to put your perceptions into the framework of knowledge you can use.

ENHANCED INTUITION - The so-called "sixth sense" is a gift we all possess. Kundalini Yoga works on your higher brain centers, and gives you the subtlety to compute the particulars of any situation, to arrive at a set of certainties you can bet on.

THE ELIMINATION OF NEGATIVE HABIT PATTERNS - Frequently we feel the need to compensate or self-destruct, due to a deep hurt or unresolved life issue. This can take the form of over-eating, drinking, drugs, and other indulgences. In the context of Kundalini Yoga there are specific techniques to help you get to the bottom of what's bothering you. In my own experience, and in the lives of my students, many negative habit patterns just fall away as a result of the applied practice of Kundalini Yoga.

RIGHT RELATIONSHIP - In our culture marriage and sexuality have lost their sacredness. In many instances "romance" simply perpetuates the particulars of a painful past. Kundalini Yoga can help you recognize and resolve your "hidden agendas."

CREATIVITY - Beyond artistic ability, creativity is a state of mind which allows you to be spontaneous, industrious, and expressive. Kundalini Yoga can help make everything you do a unique personal statement.

A HEIGHTENED SPIRITUAL SENSE - Sometime we feel like it's us against the world. Life seems to be nothing more than a never-ending attempt to pay the bills, put food on the table, and keep our cars swathed in spark plugs. Kundalini Yoga will imbue you with an expansive overview, to the extent that you begin to see of a vast and ordered framework which supports your every endeavor.

I have included this list of the general benefits of Kundalini Yoga not only to whet your appetite, but to get you thinking along certain lines. You may never have considered that any exercise or self-help system could be so comprehensive and profound.

I cannot substantiate these claims as a scientist, I can only say that time and again as a Teacher of Kundalini Yoga, I've seen people change their lives for the better, get well, and help others in turn. This is no accident. In the thousands of years in which Kundalini Yoga has been extant, it's been honed to meet the exigencies of life, for and by people just like us.

HISTORICAL OVERVIEW

We can only guess at the true age of Kundalini Yoga. It is known that over time, men and women of wisdom, through observation and experimentation, compiled a vast body of knowledge relating to health, healing, and spiritual development.

Although yogic disciplines can be found in many cultures and traditions, yoga originally coalesced and flowered in India. Traditionally yoga was broken down into stages, each of which had to be mastered before the next one could be learned.

Over time each of these stages became a system unto itself in much the same way as medicine has become compartmentalized i.e. cardiology, rheumatology, neurology, gastroenterology, dermatology, and a host of others. Many doctors and patients have lost sight of the fact that healing is an integrated process in which every facet of you must be taken into consideration.

Kundalini Yoga is called the Mother of all Yogas because it's the original system from which all other yogas stem. To increase your understanding of what Kundalini Yoga truly entails, I think it would be helpful to delineate the various stages which Kundalini Yoga encompasses.

Traditionally, before an aspirant was taught anything he/she had to adhere to a set of moral constraints. These were called *Yamas* and *Nyamas*, or do's and don'ts. These included a set of ethics and lifestyle considerations, which included respect for all life, right livelihood, and right relationship.

HATHA YOGA - *Hatha Yoga* is a system of physical exercises and poses which brings flexibility and balance to the body and being

PRANAYAM - *Pranayam* is the science of breathing. The power and profundity of conscious breathing should not be underestimated. Breathing is one of the most important tools in Kundalini Yoga. Much more about this later!

MANTRA YOGA - *Mantras* are special words or phrases of power which can help you de-stress and stay focused, clear, and inspired.

LAYA YOGA - *Laya Yoga* combines breath, *mantra*, and rhythm, to engender higher mental states. It's closely linked to *Naad Yoga* which is the science of sound vibration and its effect on your state of being.

RAJA YOGA - *Raja Yoga* combines concentration and visualization techniques to stimulate the energy centers which lie along the spine (see appendix 1) to activate your attributes and let the true you shine through.

KUNDALINI YOGA, then, is a system which utilizes exercise, breathing, the science of sound and rhythm, and the beaming power of your mind, to help you live a life in accordance with your inner aims, and arrive at an experience which is your birthright and Destiny.

Kundalini Yoga is a householder's yoga. It recognizes the fact that you need not take up residence in a monastery or cave, or wander the continents with a begging bowl, to accrue merit or find meaning in life. By simply integrating these practices into your normal routine, and doing your best to live consciously, you can go a long way in terms of personal growth, and make great gains on the inner planes.

Kundalini Yoga was first taught in the West by Yogi Bhajan, Ph.D, who in 1969, recognized that the young people in America, who were experimenting with drugs and alternative lifestyles, needed something tangible to quench their inner thirst. His decision to teach Kundalini Yoga was somewhat momentous, because it had never been taught openly before.

Yogi Bhajan contends that in this time of great transition and transformation (which many are calling the onset of the Aquarian age) secret practices and societies are no longer indicated. He feels that every person has an inherent birthright to be healthy and happy, and the means towards the realization of this is within each of us.

This book is designed to be a kind of self-help compendium. I've tried to include techniques which address the needs and concerns which engage us all. I hope that you will familiarize yourself with the contents of this book, to the extent you make the techniques part of your life.

This book is for you, whether you're in shape, out of shape, or wavering between the two. Be willing to begin slowly, step by step. In this culture of fast food, instant gratification, and glitter over substance, we tend to want dramatic results right away. Kundalini Yoga will give you results right away, but you have to be willing to patiently observe the effects, and set yourself for the long haul. This means to do your discipline every day.

Many people equate yoga with something other-worldly or exotic; they don't see its relevance to their daily lives. Don't procrastinate about beginning your yoga practice by thinking that you have to be "perfect" to begin. I've heard people say, 'Well, I think I'll wait until I move to the country before I take up yoga or meditation; I just can't concentrate in New York,' or, 'Before I take a class I want to lose ten pounds.' Start where you're at, and take it from there. Kundalini Yoga is for you to use in the context of your life, right now.

CHAPTER 1 - GETTING STARTED

GENERAL GUIDELINES

DO'S

1. Wear comfortable clothes you can move in. Natural fibers are best.

2. When at all possible do yoga in clean and accommodating environments. Remember though, that there are techniques in Kundalini Yoga which you can use anywhere, whether it be in your Dentist's waiting room, while waiting to tee off at the golf course, or in the wings before a performance.

3. It's best to do yoga barefoot so the nerve-endings in your feet can breathe.

4. Always keep your spine and shoulders covered (with a shawl, blanket, or sweater, etc.) while doing any kind of extended meditation.

5. KEEP UP! If there's a philosophy which best serves as the underpinning for this system, it's probably best summed up in these two words. In the context of an exercise, or in trying to maintain a discipline in your life, you're bound to meet resistance (as your old habits try to assert themselves). Cultivate a habit of doing more than you thought you could. This is when the real payoff comes. Also, let common sense be commensurate with your strivings.

DONT'S

1. Don't eat 2-3 hours before practicing yoga. If you're famished, something light, like a piece of fruit is okay.

2. Never practice yoga under the influence of drugs or alcohol. If you're taking medication consult your physician before proceeding.

3. Don't aggravate an existing injury. If you're creative, you can work around it and ultimately help the healing process.

TOOLS OF THE TRADE

AIR FARE - THE BREATH

Breath is more than just a grouping of elemental gases, but a conveyance for life force, or in yogic parlance- *prana*. As in the world view of the ancients, evidence of this life force can be seen in the dramatic flux of nature i.e. the wind, lightning, and in the upward thrust of the first trembling tulips of spring! Consequently, according to yoga, the more we breathe consciously, the more alive we'll be, and the longer we'll have to be so.

There's a direct correlation between the rate and depth of our breathing and mental and emotional states. You may have noticed that when you're angry, overwrought, or in a state of stress, your breathing is somewhat shallow and rapid.

Conversely, by deepening and slowing your breathing, you're able to relax and think clearly. Most people breathe about 12-16 times a minute. It's said that if you can learn to breathe consistently 8 times or less per minute. you will become powerfully intuitive and ultimately gain a greater degree of control over your inner and outer life.

Regarding the mechanics of breathing: Air is drawn in through the nostrils, and a series of progressively smaller pathways, until it enters the lungs. It is then absorbed into the bloodstream which, in turn divests itself of impurities (the by-products of the metabolic process). Oxygen is then carried by the bloodstream to the cells to keep our life processes functioning.

Conscious breathing is a way in which we can regenerate ourselves and to some extent interdict the aging process. A deep breath is a purifying wave which gives us an inner massage.

In Kundalini Yoga we do most of our breathing through the nose, unless otherwise specified. Our nose has been specifically designed by nature to filter and prepare the incoming air for easy assimilation. Overall, conscious yogic breathing will charge your body's battery. When that happens clear the roads!

BASIC BREATHING TECHNIQUES IN KUNDALINI YOGA

In Kundalini Yoga we use a few different modes of breathing each of which is most appropriate in certain contexts. As you will see, the breath to be used is indicated in the instructions accompanying each exercise. Try to familiarize yourself with the various breathing patterns, so you won't have to refer back to this section in the middle of your workout.

LONG DEEP BREATHING

Long deep breathing is a tonic for the body and mind. It's also called diaphragmatic breathing because the diaphragm expands on each inhale to let the breath fill the abdominal area. In preparation for a deep breath you must first allow yourself to be relaxed, from the face and throat, through the-pelvic floor. A deep inhale is not necessarily forceful. You simply allow the space created by your initial relaxation to fill. To breathe properly you may need to retrain yourself. In fact most people breathe with the upper third of their lungs only. Correct breathing is a very natural process. Stay relaxed and let yourself be breathed!

Lie on your back with your feet flat and knees bent. Place your hands on your diaphragm with your palms flat, and no space between the fingertips. Relax your stomach and inhale through your nose. Your fingers should separate as the abdomen expands. Exhale through your nose, pulling your navel in slightly to facilitate the complete voiding of air, so as to prepare for the next inhale. Practice this until you're able to breathe deeply without having to strain.

BREATH OF FIRE

Now we're going to learn something which dragons have been doing for years. It's called the Breath of Fire. Breath of Fire is a very important and powerful tool in Kundalini Yoga. It's a rapid rhythmic breath through the nose which puts an equal emphasis on the inhale and exhale. Breath of Fire is a shallow breath. In many ways it resembles sniffing. Even though it's a shallow breath, you'll find your navel and diaphragm moving in rhythm with the breath.

9

The traditional claims for the Breath of Fire are legion. Here are a few:

• It oxygenates the blood, so that your body can detoxify more effectively, and regenerate itself.

• It creates what's been called a phase lock or harmonic resonance, among all systems and organs. In other words, Breath of Fire creates an over-riding rhythm which all your internal rhythms adhere to. This in turn puts you in sync with yourself, and your environments.

• Breath of Fire activates thc energy flows in the body. Breath of Fire done for one minute engenders internal effects that would've taken up to an hour with normal breathing.

• When done on a regular basis, Breath of Fire will prevent the build-up of pollutants in thc lungs.

Techniques like Breath of Fire are ideal for those of us who don't have hours a day to do yoga. They give us maximum benefits in a very short time.

SEGMENTED BREATHING

This technique involves breathing in increments. There's always a specific ratio of breaths per inhale/exhale. A typical energizing breath might entail inhaling in 4 equal parts and exhaling in 4 equal parts.

Many of the exercises in Kundalini Yoga involve breathing in conjunction with specific movements. Breathe and move with vigor in a rhythmic and relaxed way.

MUDRAS

The word *mudra* means position or attitude. This usually relates to hand or body poses held during exercises or meditations. It should be understood that these particular configurations are more than symbolic. They create specific circuits in the nervous system, increase blood flow to, and stimulate certain areas of the brain, and activate energy flows.

One of the basic *mudras* in Kundalini Yoga is *Gyan Mudra*. In this hand position the thumb and index finger tips are meeting. *Gyan* means wisdom. This hand position is usually used when meditating between exercises, to help incorporate the experience the exercise gave you into the realm of your personality and projection.

WORKING ON THE MIND AS WELL AS THE BODY
"Bow to your faith, and let the conquest of your mind
become the aim of your life." -Sikh scripture

In Kundalini Yoga we want to raise the frequency of the energy we garner, so that the self-healing process can be enhanced. We also seek to clear our minds of deep-seated stress, which lessens our effectiveness and ability to seek and find fulfillment in life.

To accomplish these tasks we use what's called a *mantra*. The word *mantra* means mind protector and/or mind projector. It "jams" the broadcasts of our negativity, doubt, and fear, so as to protect us from the patterns which keep us limited.

Mantras also help our minds to become one pointed, by filtering extraneous thoughts. When our minds are focused we tend to get more done and become successful at whatever we do in life.

Mantras are more than just random syllables. They're coded sounds, each with a unique vibratory effect, which can help you find and keep your center. In addition, the meaning of each *mantra* implants a positive affirmation deep in your psyche.

11

All language in fact has *mantric* qualities. If we fall into the habit of cursing all the time, we'll no doubt begin to exhibit a coarse demeanor. Conversely if we habitually try to speak with conscious integrity, we'll be known as truthful and dependable.

To put it another way, the qualities of any given thing are determined by its rate of vibration. *Mantras* are sounds or groupings of sounds with a pre-determined vibratory effect.

The basic all-purpose *mantra* in Kundalini Yoga is *Sat Nam* (it rhymes with "but mom"). *Sat* means Truth, and *Nam* means Name or Identity. *Sat Nam* means, then, True Identity, or the highest frequency that you in essence embody. In other words, the real you, not what others think of you, what you get paid to do, your genetic patterning, cultural conditioning, or any of the other variables which to some extent describe you. These are all part of what you are, but your True Self is the permanent aspect of you that can never be compromised or detracted from.

Unless otherwise specified, you should always intone *Sat Nam* mentally during every exercise with whatever breath rhythm is indicated (on the inhale think *Sat* and on the exhale think *Nam*). Meditate as you move. This will greatly enhance the benefits of each exercise. You should also intone *Sat Nam* while relaxing or meditating between exercises.

FOCUS OF THE EYES DURING EXERCISES

Unless otherwise specified the eyes are closed during exercises. We do this to internalize and recirculate energy we'd normally be expending (have you ever noticed how tiring the simple act of looking at things can be? i.e. going to a museum or art gallery). The energy you're conserving can be used by the body and mind to enhance the self-healing process.

When you shift your eyes in specific directions, you're actually stimulating specific areas of the brain. Also, when you eyes are fixed, your mind is fixed. Conversely, when your eyes wander, your mind also wanders.

As the eyes are closed we usually have them turned up towards the brow, that is, the point between the eyebrows, a little above the bridge of the nose. Your eyes are literally crossed slightly and looking up. This may take some time to get used to but it's definitely worth the effort.

The point between the eyebrows is called the Third Eye Point, so-called, because whereas our physical eyes give us outer sight, the Third Eye, when activated, engenders intuition and insight.

The Third Eye is an energy center or *chakra* (see appendix 1) which is the etheric counterpart of the pituitary gland. In a physical sense the pituitary relates to growth factors in the body. In a metaphysical sense the pituitary has been linked to higher mental states such as euphoria, prophetic capability, and visionary experiences.

The Third Eye has been called the command center of your awareness. This relates to your ability to monitor and control thoughts. Many beginning meditators consider it a revelation that they can pick and choose which thoughts or impulses to act upon. What we term a meditative mind is your ability to make responsible decisions in the interest of your "higher self."

Other important foci of the eyes entail: gazing at the tip of the nose, with the eyes 1/10 open, and looking up and in towards the top of the head.

BASIC SAT NAM MEDITATION

Kundalini Yoga is like a gourmet buffet; there are so many delectable techniques, it's hard to know where to begin. The fact is though, you'll find yourself drawn to the sets you need at any given time. In addition, be attentive to the techniques you feel most resistance to; you probably need to do them too!

The following meditation is usually practiced between exercises to consolidate one's gains. It can also be practiced, of course, as a technique unto itself. Although simple, its benefits are powerful and profound.

Sat Nam is an example of what's called a *Bij* or seed *mantra*. This means that from the first time you say or intone it, you plant a seed in your psyche which will bear fruit and blossom, as you water it with your personal practice.

Sit with your legs crossed or in a chair with your spine straight. Your hands are in *Gyan Mudra* (thumbs and index finger tips meeting on each hand with the other fingers straight). If you're sitting with your legs crossed, the wrists are on the knees with the palms facing up.

Your eyes are closed and turned up towards the brow. Breath deep and slow through your nose. As you inhale think *Sat* and as you exhale think *Nam*. If your mind wanders bring it back. Meditate for as long as you'd like. This technique will make a definite difference in your day and in your life.

After meditating take time to stretch before resuming other activities.

BASIC BODY LOCKS

These are combinations of muscle contractions which help to consolidate and enhance the effects of Kundalini Yoga exercises and meditations. The four locks are Root Lock, Diaphragm Lock, Neck Lock, and the simultaneous use of all of them called *Maha Bhand* or Great Lock.

Root Lock or *Mul Bhand* entails the simultaneous contraction of the anal sphincter, and sex organ, while pulling the navel in towards the spine.

Diaphragm Lock is applied by pulling the diaphragm muscle up under the ribs. This is usually applied while holding the breath out only.

Neck Lock involves pulling your chin back, like a soldier at attention. Always use this when holding the breath in or out, and while meditating.

Maha Bhand as explained, is when you contract Root Lock, Diaphragm lock, and Neck Lock at the same time. This is usually done while holding the breath in or out at the end of an exercise. Be attentive to the use of these locks in Chapter 3, and employ them on your own in subsequent chapters.

THE SCIENCE OF SEQUENCE

In Kundalini Yoga we garner an effect greater than the sum of the parts. Any exercise or set which fulfills this requirement is called a *kriya*. The literal meaning of the word *kriya* is completed action.

Each set in Kundalini Yoga works on many levels simultaneously, and has been formulated with the recognition of the working relationship between the various systems that comprise us. Kundalini Yoga sees the body/mind as a holographic construct, meaning that each part contains the whole.

RELAXATION

In Kundalini Yoga we relax between exercises so the work we've done can work for us. We want to give ourselves time for our body/mind to process the process, and make use of the energy garnered in furtherance of self-healing and balance.

In addition, relaxing between exercises will give you the ability to relax between the activities of your daily life. There's an ethic in our culture which has been misunderstood to mean that unless you're doing something all the time you're somehow non-productive. It's important to realize that conscious relaxation is doing something in the true sense of the word do!

15

Believe it or not, relaxation may be one of the hardest exercises in this book! Many of the most ostensibly successful people are totally unable to relax.. Like any other skill, it takes practice. Most of us have placed relaxation last on our list of priorities. Make conscious relaxation a part of your life.

If not specifically designated that you move on immediately, relax on your back after every one to three exercises. Unless otherwise specified, you can also meditate on *Sat Nam* while sitting in easy pose (a comfortable cross-legged position) at those times between exercises when you're not relaxing on your back.

TUNING IN

We begin every Kundalini Yoga class or practice session by chanting a special mantra. This is for protection and guidance, and to help us tune into the part of us which wants to grow and expand. The mantra is:

Ong Namo Guru Dev Namo

Its literal translation is: Infinite Creative Consciousness *(Ong)*, I call on you *(Namo)*, Divine Wisdom within *(Guru Dev)*, I call on you *(Namo)*.
It's chanted with the hands in Prayer Pose, that is, palms together, thumbs against the sternum. We do it 3 times (see below).

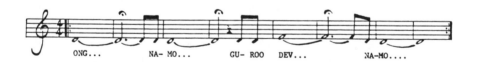

Inhale deeply through the nose and chant *Ong* (very nasal) *Namo*, then take a quick inaudible breath through the mouth, and chant *Guru Dev Namo*.

It's chanted in a monotone except for the syllable *Dev* which is a minor third higher than the tonic. You may not initially understand the relevance of using this *mantra* to begin your sessions. As with any other new endeavor, sometimes a leap of faith is required. In time though, you'll begin to appreciate the beauty of this subtle science. If circumstances don't allow you to do this out loud, you can repeat it mentally.

In its ability to help us contact our creative source, *Ong Namo Guru Dev Namo*, can help you any time inspiration is in order, whether it entails writing a poem, meeting a new client, or making dinner for someone special. It's also to very useful when you're feeling confused or seek guidance.

THE CHAKRAS

Yoga has provided some very useful models which give us cogent insights into human psychology and potential. One of these is a system of energy centers called the *chakras*.

These are locuses of energy which correspond to nerve plexi or glands. Each *chakra* has a specific quality or frequency which relates to aspects of our personality and predilections. (See appendix 1 for a more detailed description of the *chakras*.)

One way in which Kundalini Yoga transforms us, lies in its ability to insure the free flow of energy through the *chakras*. In this sense it's a kind of alchemy. We want to transform the lead of the lower self into the gold of the higher, and thus turn greed into giving, lust into desire to be higher, and anger into inspiration.

According to yoga, and many other disciplines, unless we take matters into our own hands, we're subject to entropy, that is a downward spiral. It's not hard to forget that there's more to our existence than food, sex, status, and survival. Through Kundalini Yoga we want to be grounded and aware, with faith in the fact that the Unseen is ultimately more powerful than the seen.

17

Exclamation of Ecstasy

My old self is a widow;
I died in the war of the worlds
And climbed the ladder on fire.
Patterns and persuasions were rungs
Sacrificed for my ascension.

The windmills of the heart
Grind the grain of life's lessons
And fling blazing suns and moons
Into the dormitory of the sky.

I am in love with my soul
And the Soul of all souls.
The Physician who cures me
Is the compass of the lonely.

I read a library and thought I knew Wisdom
But now I know I know nothing
And my head bows to my heart
So my apprenticeship can finally start.

O Lover of the Ocean whose breath is the wind,
Author of the Mysteries
Whose order Kings cannot rescind.
"My eyes demand to be fed on your Beauty."

I am a sub-private in the army of your novitiates.
I'd be a Times Square whore if I knew you'd select me.
I'd give my lives' savings to be a crumb on your floor.

--Ravi Singh

CHAPTER 2 - HOW TO USE THIS BOOK

Many of the exercise sequences in this book are relatively short, 15-30 minutes. This makes them especially suitable for the busiest of schedules.

As with any other activity which requires your time and effort, a consistent yoga practice takes discipline. Eventually though, you'll probably find that it's a lot harder not to do the yoga! It becomes a positive addiction which will serve you for a lifetime.

In the beginning, whatever you can do is fine. It takes most students a while before their personal practice can match the intensity of a group class.

In fact, if you haven't done so already, I strongly recommend that you seek out a Kundalini Yoga (see appendix 4) class in your area. Working with a qualified instructor will insure that you're doing the yoga correctly, and give you a chance to ask any questions you may have.

Once you get a feeling for Kundalini Yoga, you'll probably find yourself wanting to do more. Most serious practitioners do 45 minutes - 1 hour of yoga, once or twice a day, in addition to an extended meditation following the yoga.

When you become familiar with this book you can do some warm-up exercises, a sequence from one of the chapters, and a meditation (as outlined in the specific chapters or in Chapter 21).

For self-maintenance, and to be properly prepared to work on ourselves, certain things need to get covered every day. These include: flexing the spine, stretching the life (sciatic) nerve, centering and activating the Navel Center, and recharging the Magnetic Field. Try to supplement the set you practice with these types of exercises.

Although sensitivity and instinct will usually lead you in the right direction, when combining warm-up exercises, it's best not to take too many liberties until you consult a qualified Kundalini Yoga Teacher.

So, the ultimate purpose of Kundalini Yoga is to help you attain and maintain higher consciousness. This is not something you go after once and then rest easy. It's an exercise that lasts a lifetime.

Spirit rising-
Engine of my soul,
Between you and I
There is a moment
When the self becomes whole,
Breath overthrows death,
And opposites salute the other
In Infinity's deep embrace.

By your Grace,
White wisdom fills my being,
And I hear songs of praise the Universe sings.

--Ravi Singh

CHAPTER 3 - BEGINNERS' SETS

The following introductory sets are effective daily maintenance regimes. When yoga's the last thing you feel like doing, you probably need it the most. These sequences can help you go about your day in a great way.

BEGINNERS' SET # 1

1. With your hands in prayer pose (palms pressed together thumbs against the sternum), tune in with: *Ong Namo Guru Dev Namo*

Keep your hands in Prayer Pose and take 15 complete, deep breaths through your nose. Then do Breath of Fire for 1-2 minutes. (figure 1) Inhale (apply Neck Lock), hold the breath and contract the muscles of the rectum, sex organ, and navel point (Root Lock). After 5-10 seconds exhale completely and hold the breath out for 5-10 seconds, squeezing Root Lock. Inhale, then relax the breath and meditate. Inhale think, *Sat* and as you exhale think *Nam*. Consolidate your gains. Continue meditating for 1-2 minutes, then proceed to the next exercise.

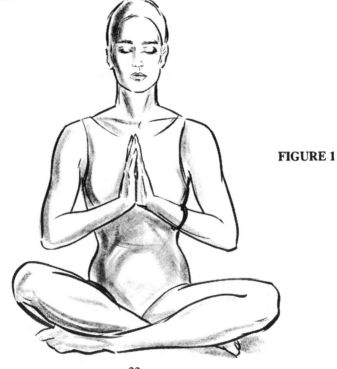

FIGURE 1

2. Extend your arms out to the sides and raise them to a 60 degree angle. The palms face inward (figure 2). Do the Breath of Fire for 1-3 minutes. Inhale, hold the breath and apply Root Lock, exhale, hold the breath out and squeeze up, inhale, relax the breath, let the arms float down to the sides, like the wings of a white great bird, having attained the sacred summit.

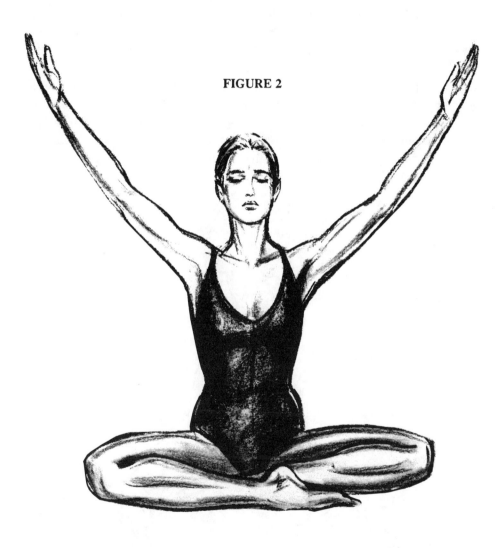

FIGURE 2

3. This one's called Camel Ride. Sit with your legs crossed and hold your shins (figure 3). As you inhale press your lower spine forward, and as your exhale flex it back (figure 4) Use your hands and arm strength somewhat to facilitate the flex. The speed of this exercise is up to you. It can be done with some rapidity.

Throughout the exercise keep your diaphragm relaxed, your face facing forward, and your head in line with the spine. Continue rhythmically for 1-3 minutes. To end inhale and straighten up and squeeze Root Lock with the breath held in and out. Then relax the breath and meditate for 1-2 minutes.

4. Still sitting with your legs crossed, place your hands on your shoulders with your fingers in front, thumbs in back. As you inhale twist to the left, and as you exhale twist to the right (figure 5). The movement is continuous. Maintain your focus at the brow point (the Third Eye). Keep going for 1-3 minutes. To end pull Root Lock with the breath held and expelled.

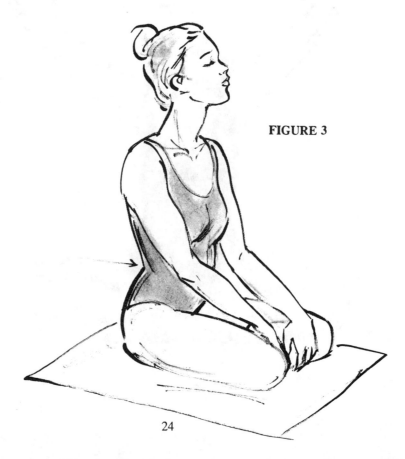

FIGURE 3

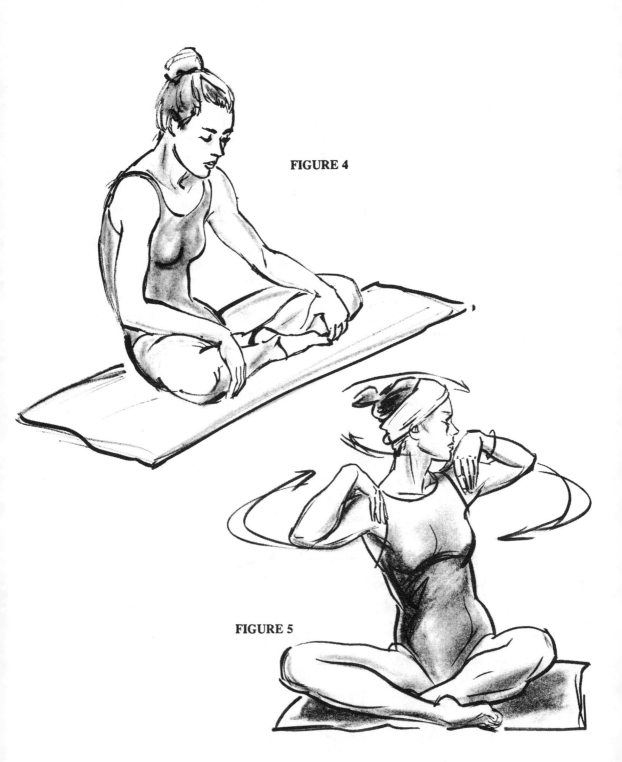

FIGURE 4

FIGURE 5

25

5. Relax on your back with your arms by your sides, palms facing up. Let the work you've done thus far work for you now. (figure 6)

6. Remain on your back. Have your knees bent and feet flat. Your arms are by your sides with your palms facing down. Press your hips up so that your lower back clears the ground. Do Breath of Fire and continue for 1-2 minutes (figure 7). Inhale deep and relax, with your legs extended, for about 1-2 minutes. Then wrap your arms around your knees and rock and roll on your spine.

7. Lie on your back again. As you inhale raise your right arm and left leg straight up, and exhale as you lower them. Then inhale as your raise your left arm and right leg straight up and exhale as you lower them (figure 8). Continue these alternate leg and arm raises to and from ninety degrees, for 2-5 minutes. Then relax on your back.

FIGURE 6

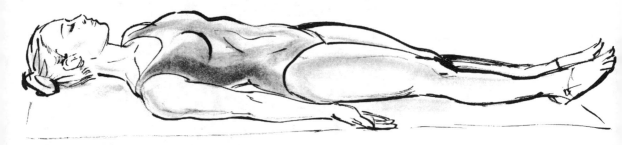

FIGURE 7

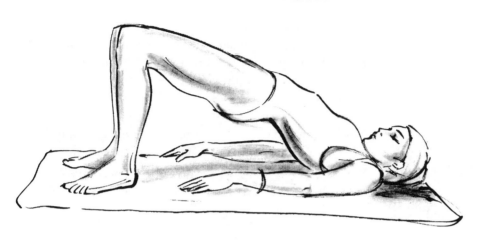

FIGURE 8

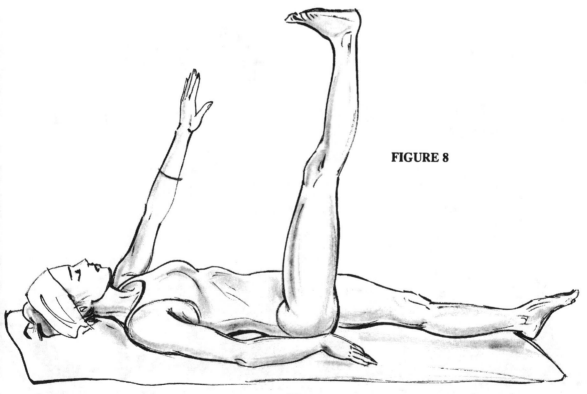

8. Again wrap your arms around your bent knees, tuck your nose and rock on your spine (figure 9).

9. Sit on your heels in Rock Pose (if this is not possible for you, sit with your legs crossed and hold your knees). Your hands are on your thighs, palms facing down. As you inhale flex your spine forward (figure 10), and as you exhale flex back (figure 11). Continue for 1-3 minutes, then squeeze Root Lock with the breath held and expelled.

10. Sit with your legs crossed. Inhale swing your arms up (figure 11), palms facing back. Exhale swing your arms back (figure 12), inhale cross your arms in front of you, parallel to the ground, and exhale swing your arms back (figure 12). The movement is: <u>up</u>, <u>back</u>, <u>cross</u>, <u>back</u>. Do this at a good pace with a powerful breath for 2-3 minutes.   Relax.

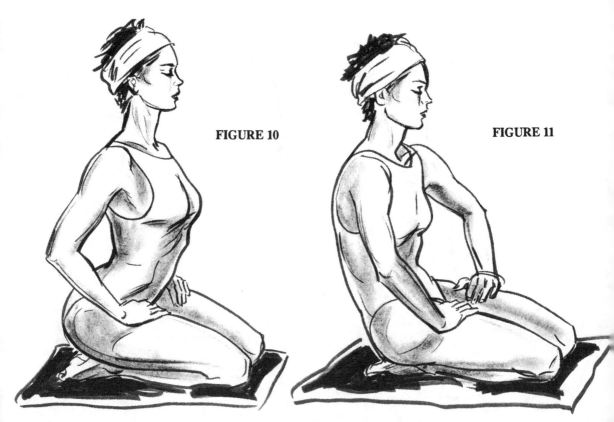

FIGURE 10

FIGURE 11

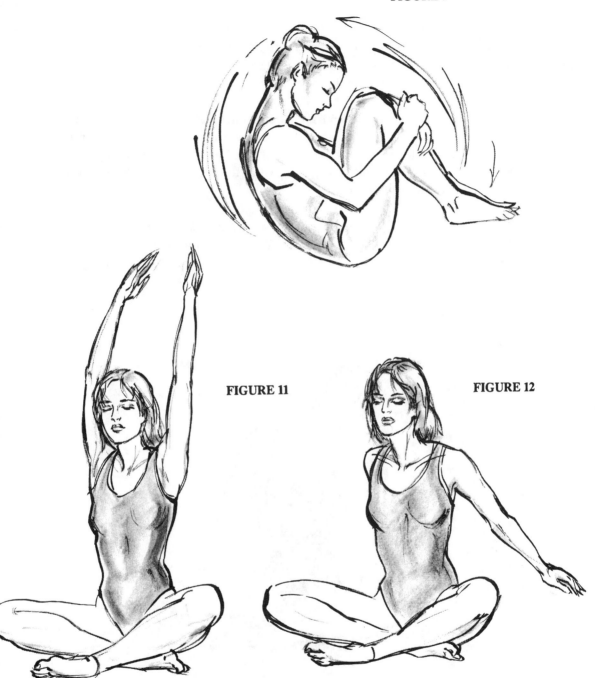

FIGURE 9

FIGURE 11

FIGURE 12

11. Neck Rolls. Sit with your legs crossed and roll your head around. Follow the course of your collarbone, taking 8-10 seconds for each rotation. Go ten times in one direction and ten in the other (figure 13).

12. Please be on your hands and knees. This one's called Cat/Cow. As you inhale press your head up and stomach down (figure 14). As you exhale curve your spine and lower your head (figure 15). Keep your elbows straight throughout the exercise and your gaze fixed at the brow point. Continue at a moderate pace for 1-3 minutes.

Cat/Cow works on every one of the 72,000 nerves which run from, to, or through the spine. It will give you total flexibility of the spine. It stimulates the optic nerve to give you sparkling eyes. It's even good to dry your hair after a shower!

FIGURE 13

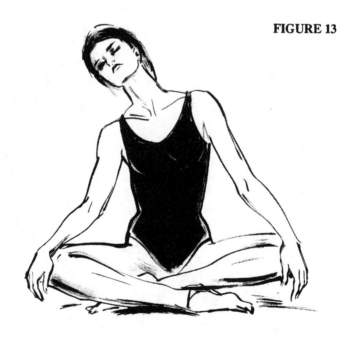

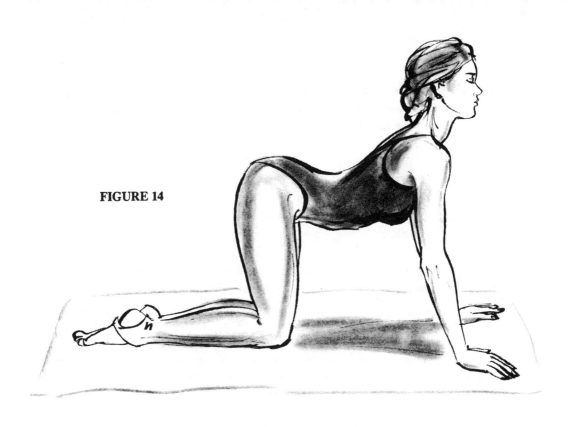

FIGURE 14

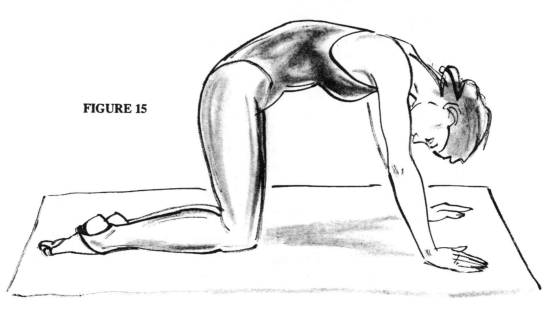

FIGURE 15

31

13. This exercise is called *Sat Kriya*. Sit on your heels if possible, otherwise have your legs crossed. Extend your arms straight up, so that the upper arms are next to your ears. Your fingers are interlaced, with the index fingers extended (figure 16).

Say the sound *Sat* as you pull your navel point in. Say the sound *Nam* as you relax your navel point. The only movement here is your stomach as it moves in and out. Keep your elbows straight throughout. Continue for 3 minutes and relax on your back.

Mentally pulsate *Sat* at the navel, and feel *Nam* rise up the spine. When you bring your mind to an exercise you greatly enhance its benefits.

Sat Kriya is one of the basic exercises in Kundalini Yoga. It massages the internal organs, helps the heart, and releases energy which is often bottled up in the lower centers. According to yoga this can help you to resolve phobias, insecurities, obsessions, and mental aberrations, since these imbalances are always associated with the lower three centers.

Sat Kriya can be practiced as an exercise unto itself. Because of its wide range of benefits it constitutes an important self-help therapy. Always remember to relax on your back equal to the time of the exercise.

Relax on your back
Like a white cloud in a blue sky
Above the hurry
And worry of the world.
Let before and later
No longer matter.
Let your body go,
Your spirit rise.
Relax & realize
That you are an essence in essence,
Inviolable & pure.
Be more relaxed than you ever were.

FIGURE 16

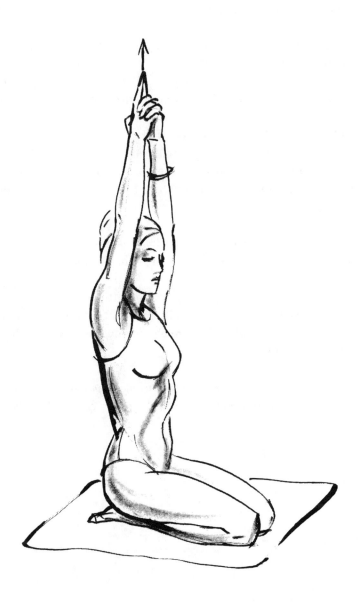

BEGINNERS' SET #2

1. Your hands are in Prayer Pose. Tune in with *Ong Namo Guru Dev Namo.*

2. Stand up. Your arms are straight up, so that your upper arms are hugging your ears. Hook your thumbs (figure 1). As you inhale lean back, and as you exhale come forward bringing your hands to or towards the ground (figure 2). Continue for 1-2 minutes. If this one's uncomfortable bend your knees.

3. Still standing. This one's called Archer Pose. Begin with your feet a little more than shoulder width apart, with your toes pointing forward. Turn your right foot to the right, and press the heel of the left foot 3 inches to the left. Bend your right knee so that your right thigh is almost parallel to the floor (figure 3).

Bend your left elbow so that the left hand is next to the left ear, in a fist. Your right arm is extended straight, parallel to the ground.

Your eyes are open gazing straight ahead. Breath long and deeply through your nose. Willingly put yourself under pressure. Continue Long Deep Breathing for 1-3 minutes, then inhale deeply, and switch sides. Relax as you stand for a minute.

This exercise is for your nerves. We want to put ourselves under pressure so as to release the deeper pressure that the stress of a lifetime has imposed

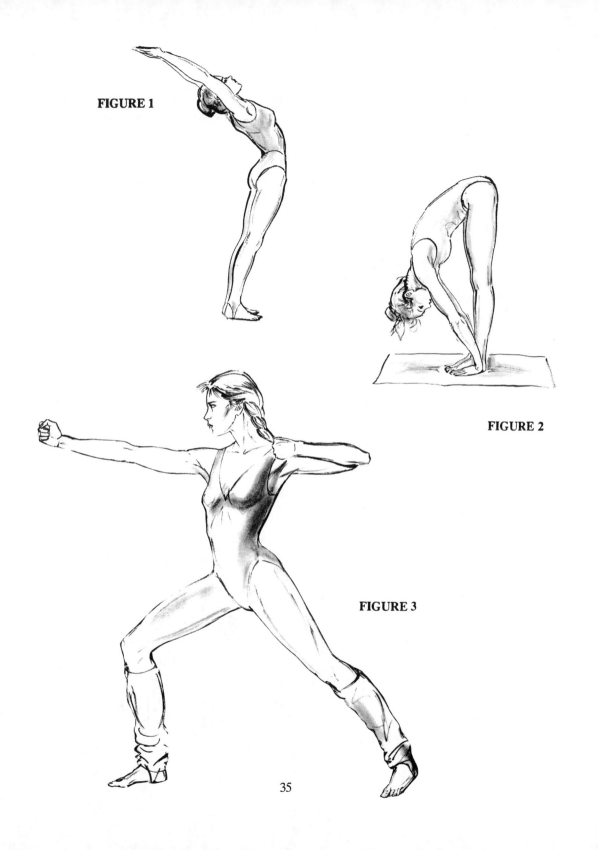

FIGURE 1

FIGURE 2

FIGURE 3

4. This one's called Frog Pose. Come into a squatting position so that your heels are together and off the ground. Your arms are between your knees, elbows straight, fingertips on the ground. (figure 4).

As you inhale straighten your knees and lower your head (figure 5). As you exhale return to the starting position. Keep your elbows straight throughout the exercise. Continue up to 26 times. Proceed immediately to the next exercise.

5. Sit on the floor with your legs extended straight. Your arms are parallel to the ground, with your fingers pointing forward and thumbs pointing up. As you inhale lean back 30 degrees, and as you exhale lean forward 30 degrees. Continue with powerful breathing for 1-3 minutes (figure 6).

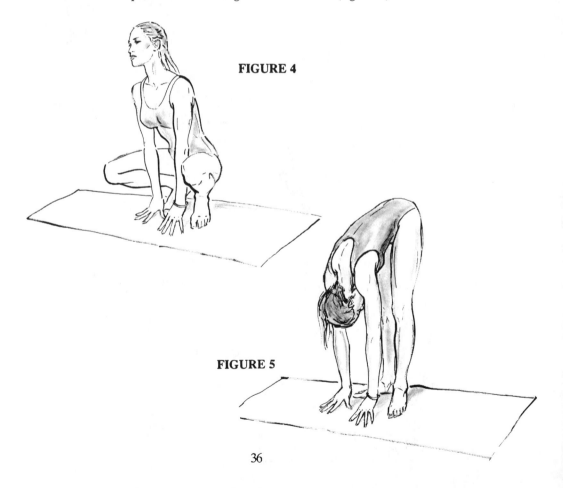

FIGURE 4

FIGURE 5

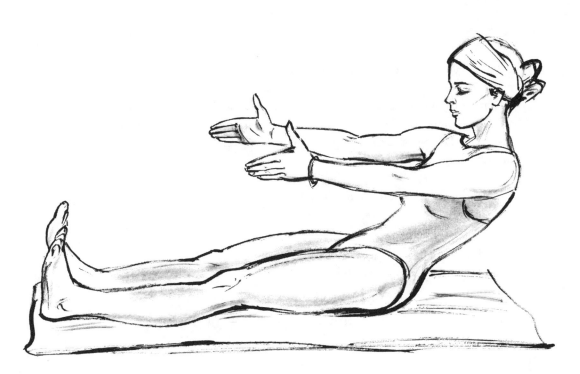

FIGURE 6

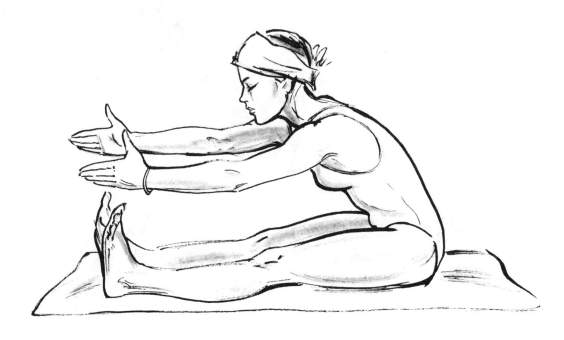

6. Relax on your back for 2 to 3 minutes.

7. Come onto your hands and knees. As you inhale raise your right arm and left leg. Exhale and return them to the starting position. Then inhale and raise your left am and right leg, and exhale lower them (figure 7). Continue for 1-3 minutes.

8. Relax on your back for a minute.

FIGURE 7

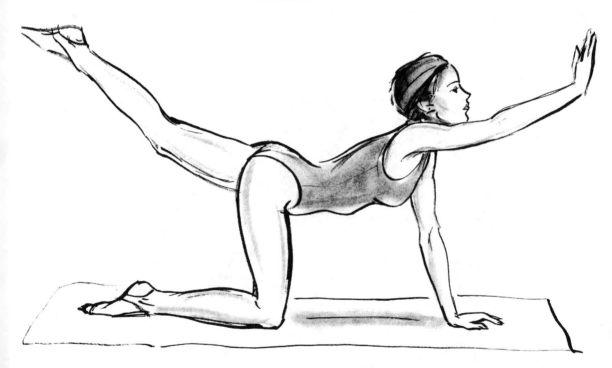

9. Sit up with your legs still extended. Support yourself with your hands. As you inhale raise your right leg, and exhale as you lower it. Then inhale raise your left leg and exhale as you lower it. Continue these alternate leg lifts for 1-3 minutes. Feel that you're funnelling breath (and thus energy) in through the navel, as you simultaneously focus at the brow, allowing *Sat Nam* and the breath to blend (figure 8).

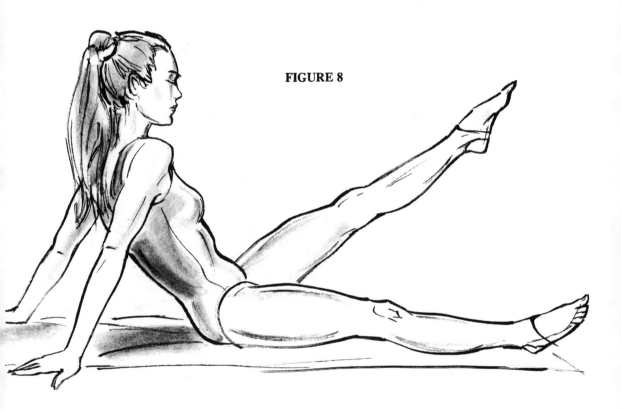

FIGURE 8

10. Lie on your stomach, with your hands under your shoulders as if you were going to do a push-up. As you inhale raise your upper body into Cobra Pose (figure 9). As you exhale lower yourself to the ground. Continue slowly for 1-2 minutes.

11. On your back again, have your hands under your buttocks for support, palms facing down. Raise your head and heels six inches, stare at your toes. This is Stretch Pose. Do Breath of Fire for 1 minute. (figure 10) Relax.

12. Wrap your arms around your knees and rock on your spine.

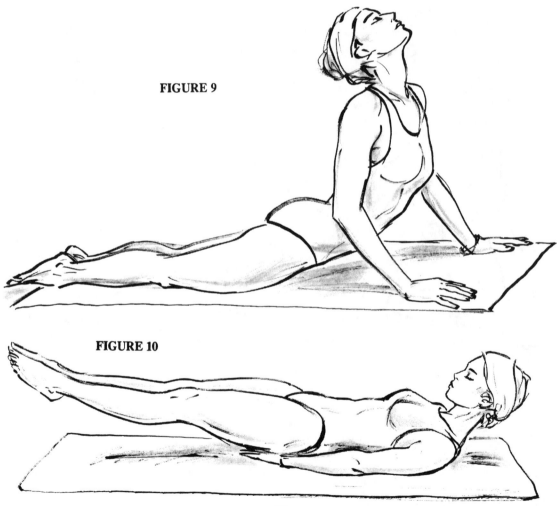

FIGURE 9

FIGURE 10

13. Sit with your legs crossed in easy pose. Extend your arms straight out to either side, with the arms parallel to the floor. Your hands are in fists with the index fingers extended. Rotate your arms in small circles backwards, in concert with the Breath of Fire. (figure 11).

Continue for 1 minute, then inhale and hold the breath. Hook your index fingers in front of the sternum and pull hard for 15 seconds. Now relax the breath, lower the arms, and meditate. Repeat the same exercise 3 more times: first with the middle finger, then the ring finger , and finally with the little finger extended.

After doing Breath of Fire, remember to inhale, hold the breath, and hook the fingers you had extended in front of the sternum, pulling apart. As you hold the breath apply Root Lock, as well as Neck Lock.

14. Lie on your back and relax.

FIGURE 11

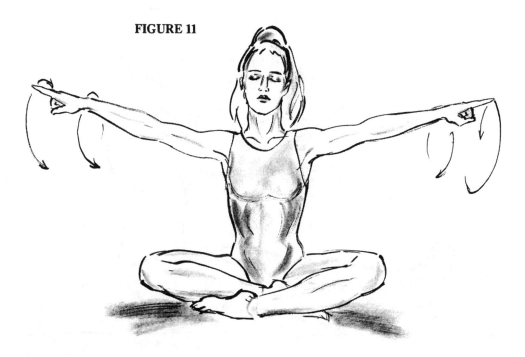

BEGINNERS' SET #3

The following brief sequence, like all Kundalini Yoga classes, can help you attain a new perspective on your problems, and make you positive.

1. Sitting with a straight spine, extend your legs straight and your arms parallel to the ground, shoulder width apart. The palms are facing down (figure 1). As you inhale lean back and raise your legs 2 feet off the ground. Exhale and come back to the original position (figure 2). Move as one unit, at a moderate pace, for 5 minutes. Inhale, relax the breath and proceed to the next exercise.

2. With your legs still in front of you, hold onto your toes (figure 3). If this isn't possible, hold your ankles. Stretch steadily for 10 minutes. Stay vigilant. To end inhale, then exhale and stretch even more. Do this 2 more times then slowly come up.

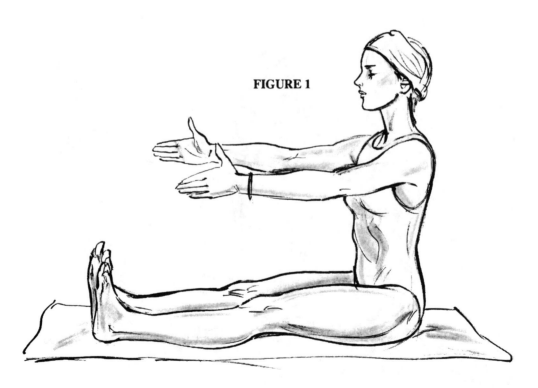

FIGURE 1

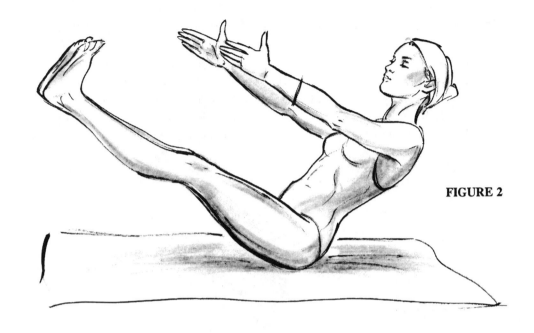

FIGURE 2

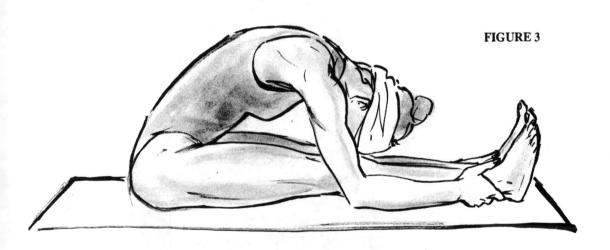

FIGURE 3

3. Sit on your heels in Rock Pose with your palms facing down on your thighs. If this is too uncomfortable sit with your legs crossed with your hands on your knees. Flex your spine (figure 4) as you whisper *Sat Nam* (*Sat* forward, *Nam* back). You can increase your rhythm steadily as you go. Continue for 8 minutes then straighten up and take 3 deep breaths. Inhale again and hold, as you apply Root Lock. Exhale, hold out and apply Root Lock. Inhale deep, relax the breath and meditate before resuming normal activities.

FIGURE 4

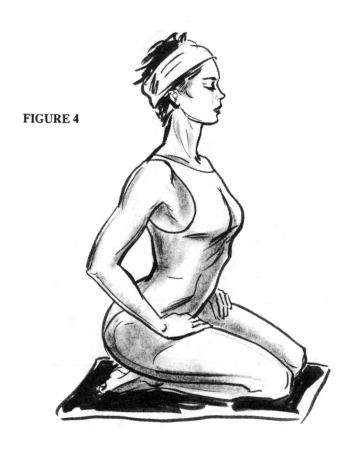

CHAPTER 4 - O MY HEALTHY BACK

Back problems abound in our culture. Many chronic back conditions can be traced to one or all of the following: improper posture, soft beds, lack of exercise, restrictive footwear such as high heels, a high stress level, unhealthy diet and nutritional deficiencies, structural mis-alignment, and emotional holding patterns. Yogic techniques and lifestyle considerations address themselves to all of these.

Ponder this equation: You're as flexible as your spine is flexible, and as young as your spine is flexible. As your spine gets progressively less pliant, with the onset of old age, it gets harder to move, and to involve yourself in the activities you once enjoyed. Also, there's a correlation between a stiff spine, and the inability to consider new experiences and possibilities.

The spine is also the housing for the central nervous system and a conveyance for Kundalini, the energy of spirit rising.

My experience as a Teacher has shown me that a high percentage of back problems seem to stem from emotional tendencies which a person harbors in his/her musculature. Psychologically speaking, the lower back is the most vulnerable part of us. For this reason many peoples' backs seize up when fear and lack of trust remain unresolved issues.

Proper breathing is an important step in learning to use the back correctly. An intractable diaphragm muscle makes proper breathing difficult. The muscles of the diaphragm encircle the torso. When the diaphragm is tight, then the upper, lower back, and hips all must compensate when you move or stretch.

True flexibility begins with a pliant spine and relaxed diaphragm and extends to the extremities.

Your kidneys and adrenals frequently bear the brunt of stressful living. When this happens your lower back will feel somewhat painful and stiff. Remember your body isn't out to get revenge on you. It's only transmitting messages to help you understand and act upon prevailing conditions. If any kind of back problem persists or is causing you pain, please see a qualified health practitioner.

The following exercises can make your spine more flexible, and help your posture. They also help create an upward momentum of energy, and cerebral-spinal fluid, towards the brain and higher centers.

1. Lie on your back. Bend your knees and cross your ankles (figure 1). Move your knees to and from the head in small movements. 1 minute.

2. Sit on your heels. Have your hands on the floor in front of your knees, palms facing down. Flex your lower spine. Inhale forward (figure 2) exhale back (figure 3) 26X.

FIGURE 1

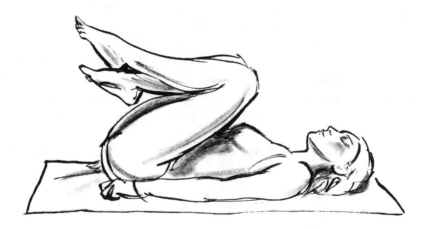

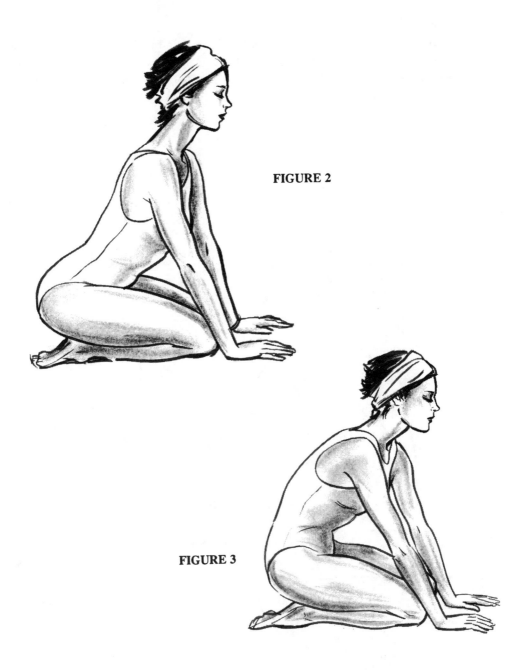

FIGURE 2

FIGURE 3

3. Extend your legs in front of you. Inhale, exhale bend your right knee and twist to the right (figure 3). Inhale, and exhale as you twist left. Keep your sit-bones on the ground. Use the cross arm as a lever and the back hand as an anchor. 1-3 minutes.

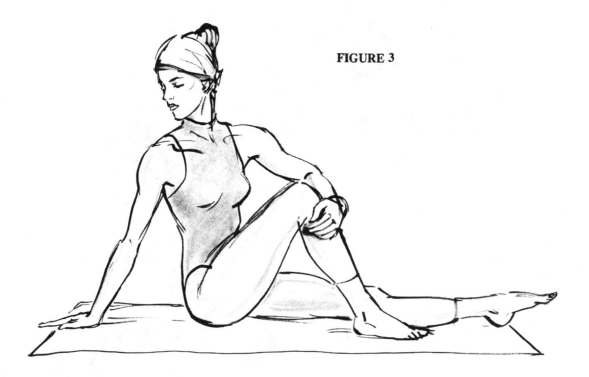

FIGURE 3

Variation: Sit with your legs crossed. Inhale and exhale as you bring your right elbow to the left knee. Inhale rise up, and exhale as you bring your left elbow to your right knee. Continue for 1 minute (figure 4)

4. Relax on your back for one minute, then wrap you your bent knees and rock and roll on your spine.

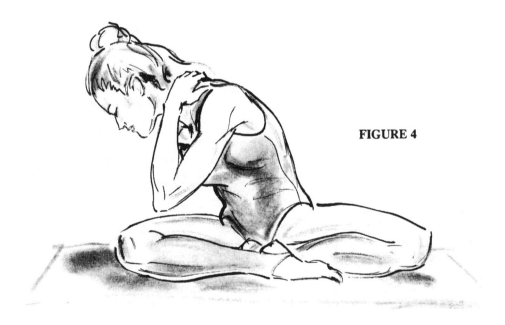

FIGURE 4

5. Lie on your stomach. Make fists around your thumbs and place your fists in the cavity formed where the thighs meet the body. Your chin is on the floor, your face facing forward.

As you inhale raise your left leg off the ground. Exhale as you lower it. Then inhale raise your right leg off the ground and exhale as you lower it (figure 5). Continue these alternate leg lifts for 1-2 minutes.

6. Lie on your back, wrap your arms around your bent knees. As you inhale extend your legs straight, at a 45 degree angle in relation to the ground (figure 7). As you exhale pull your knees into your body (figure 8). Continue for 3 minutes. Relax.

FIGURE 5

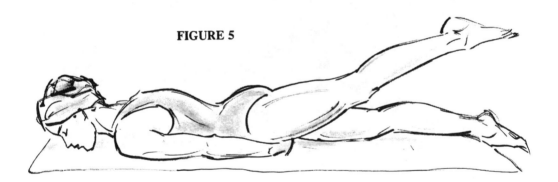

FIGURE 7

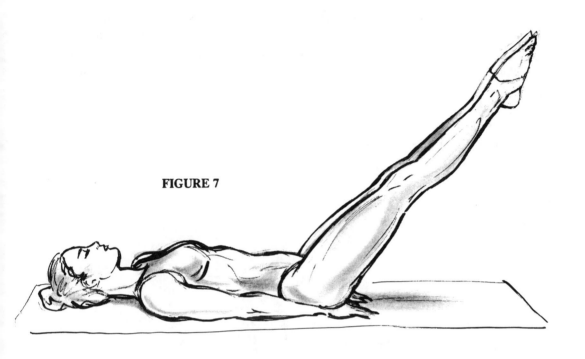

FIGURE 8

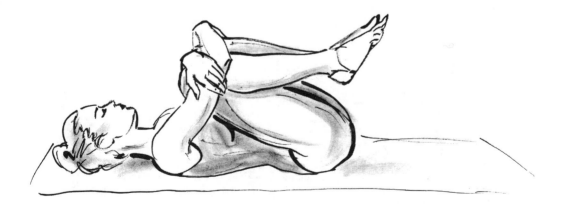

51

7. Interlace your fingers at the small of your back. Keep your hands and arms off your back through the entire exercise. As you inhale rise off your heels, press your hips forward, and arch your spine (figure 9). As you exhale sit on your heels and lower your forehead to the ground (figure 10). Continue this sequence for 1-3 minutes.

8. Relax on your back for 1-3 minutes. Then, wrap your arm your knees, tuck your nose and rock and roll on your spine.

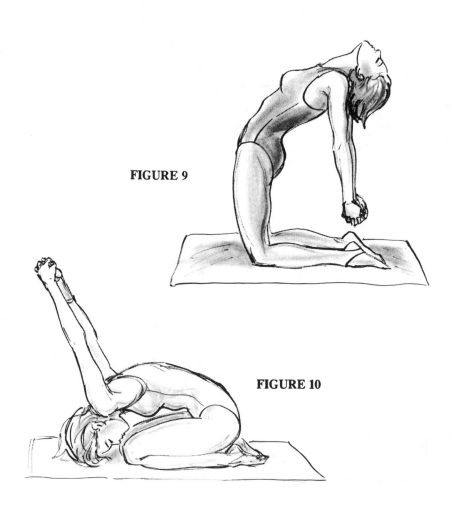

FIGURE 9

FIGURE 10

9. Sit with your legs crossed, hands on the shoulders, fingers in front, thumbs in back. As you inhale press your elbows and head back (figure 11), as you exhale lower your elbows, drop your head forward, and round your upper spine (figure 12). Continue at a good pace 1-3 minutes.

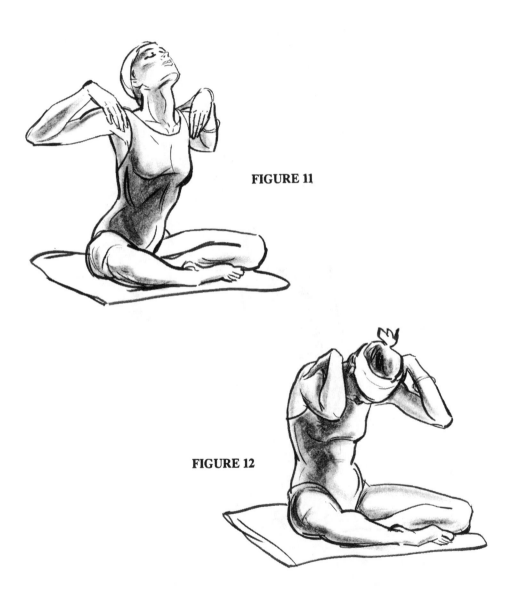

FIGURE 11

FIGURE 12

53

10. Sit cross-legged. Stretch your arms straight up so that your upper arms are hugging your ears. Your palms face inward and the fingers are very wide. Actively stretch for up to 3 minutes (figure 13). Inhale deeply and stretch up, then let the breath go and relax your hands in your lap. Meditate for 30 seconds and proceed.

Repeat the exercise for 3 -5 minutes.

11. Meditate. Inhale think *Sat* and exhale think *Nam*. Continue for as long as you'd like.

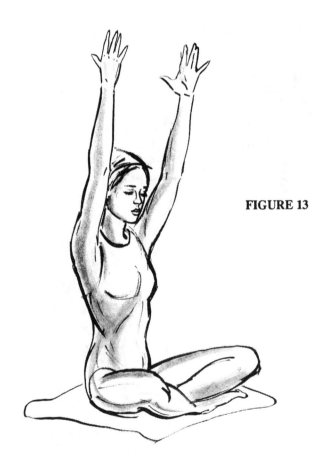

FIGURE 13

CHAPTER 5 - FLEXIBLE AND FREE

The body we show the world is a map, which depicts the landscape of our emotional tendencies. In early childhood responses to initial conditioning and environments were encoded into our musculature and very often remain permanent traits of our personality and body type.

For instance, an overabundance of tension in the shoulders has been associated with unresolved anger and resentment in the face of responsibility. Tightness in the backs of the legs has been linked with fear of flying (open to new experiences), a need to grip the earth.

We take on the qualities of whatever pose we assume. If we stand tall and walk with majesty, then these attributes will become a permanent part of our character.

While stretching allow yourself to relax through areas of tension. Be especially attentive to your breathing. Conscious breathing helps you massage your body from within and unravel the tightness a lifetime of accumulated stress has wrought.

Be systematic and set yourself for the long haul. Successful stretching entails daily practice and sensitivity to your body's particular responses. As always, if you feel any kind of pain or strain, beyond what's prudent, modify the exercise. If no relief is forthcoming, consult a qualified health practitioner.

Be like a young tree
In the breeze
Of the breath,
In the eternal spring
Of your burgeoning.

1. Standing. Your feet are 3 inches apart with the toes pointing forward. Your arms are extended straight out to the sides with the palms facing out, fingers pointing up. Bend your knees so that you feel a stretch in your shins. (figure 1). Maintain a consistent stretch in your arms also. Breath long and deeply through your nose. 1-3 minutes.

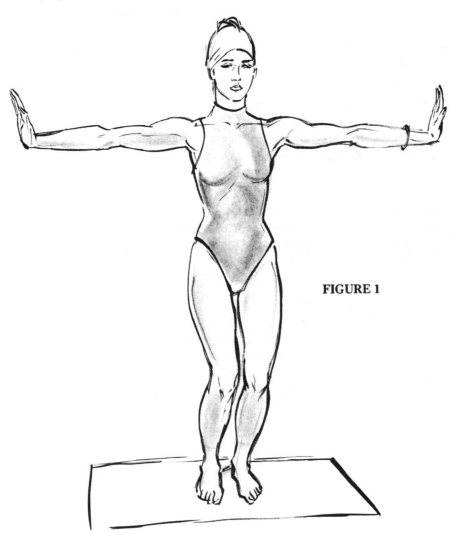

FIGURE 1

2. Extend your left leg back with the top of the foot on floor. The right knee is bent, the left thigh parallel to the ground, and your arms straight with the palms pressed together (figure 2). Stare straight and do the Breath of Fire for 1-3 minutes. Switch sides and repeat.

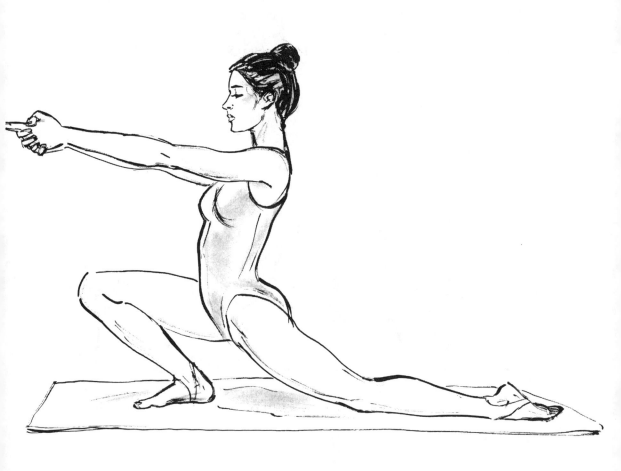

FIGURE 2

3. Sit on the floor with your legs in front of you. The sole of the left foot is pressing the inside of the right thigh, as high as it will go. Stretch down over the right leg holding onto the right foot or ankle (figure 3). Hold this pose with a normal breath for 1-3 minutes. Switch sides and repeat.

4. Sit on your right heel, with the left leg extended straight. Interlace your fingers, invert your hands, and extend your arms up so the upper arms are framing the head (figure 4). Inhale. Exhale and stretch down over the extended leg (figure 5). Continue for 1-3 minutes. Switch sides and repeat.

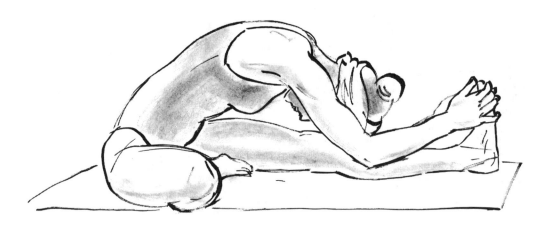

FIGURE 3

FIGURE 4

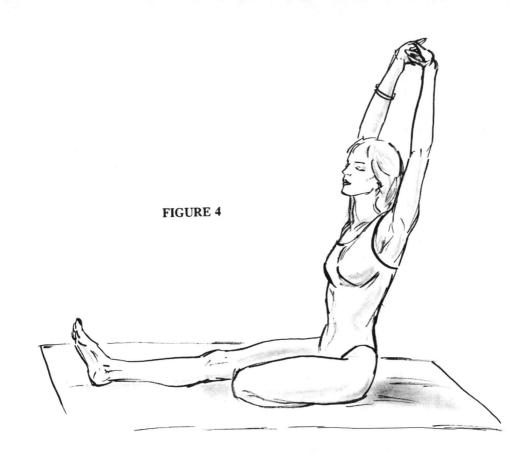

FIGURE 5

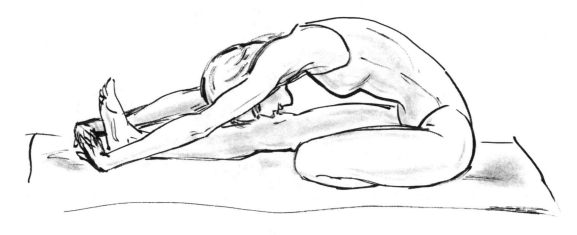

5. Now have the soles of the feet together, with the knees bent. Hold onto the feet with both hands. Use your elbows as levers against the inner calves. Now angle forward so that you feel a consistent stretch in your inner thighs. Breathe deeply and consciously. As you relax into the stretch, go a little further forward. (figure 6). 1-3 minutes.

6. Your legs are in front of you wide. Hold onto your insteps or heels. Stretch forward, bringing your sternum towards the ground. (figure 7) If this is not possible hold onto opposite elbows. Long Deep Breathing 1-3 minutes.

7. Your legs are still in front of you wide apart. Inhale up and exhale down alternating sides (figure 8). Continue at a good pace for 1-3 minutes.

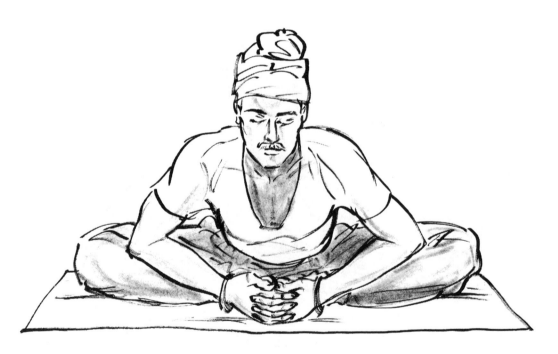

FIGURE 6

60

FIGURE 7

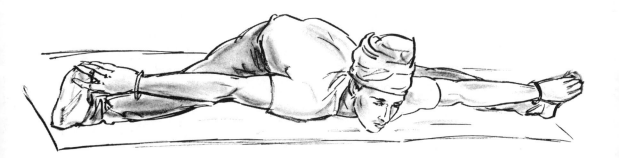

FIGURE 8

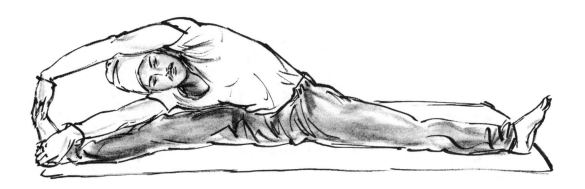

8. Lie on your back with your feet flat and knees bent. Hold onto your ankles. If this is not possible have your hands by your sides, palms down. As you inhale press your hips up, and as you exhale lower your lower back to the floor (figure 9). 26X

9. Still on your back. Inhale, then exhale as you move your legs up and over, to or towards the floor behind you (figure 10). Inhale as you lower your legs to the floor, then exhale as you sit up, grab your toes and bring your nose towards your knees (figure 11). Don't start one movement until you've completed the one before. 26X

FIGURE 9

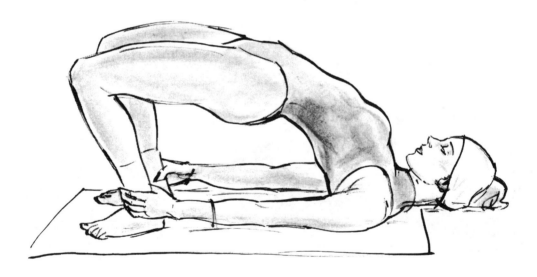

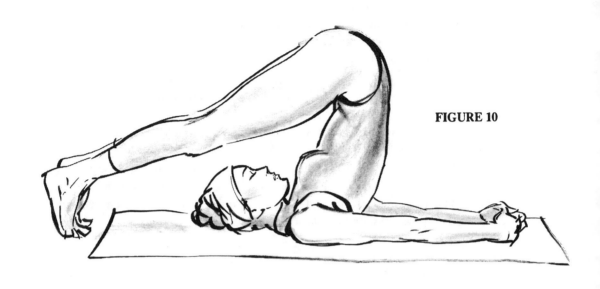

FIGURE 10

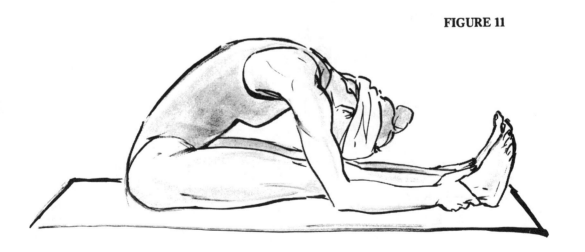

FIGURE 11

63

10. Please be on your hands and knees in Cow Pose. Keep your head up throughout the exercise. As you inhale press your stomach towards the ground (figure 12), and as you exhale pull your stomach away from the ground. Continue this spine flex at a moderate to fast pace for 1-3 minutes. Maintain the pose. Open your eyes and gaze fixedly at a point on the ceiling. Do Breath of Fire for 1-3 minutes. Immediately proceed to the next exercise.

11. Remaining on your hands and knees. Come into Cat Pose. Your spine is rounded and your head is down (figure 13). Inhale. Now exhale completely and hold the breath out. With the breath completely expelled pump your stomach vigorously. When you absolutely cannot hold the breath out inhale deep. Exhale immediately and begin pumping again. When you've completed 8 cycles sit with your legs crossed, and meditate.

This exercise will add to your flexibility by helping to open your solar plexus which in turn will enable you to move and bend easily and breathe deeply and effortlessly, In addition this technique helps your heart, digestive system, and will help your adrenals recover from long term stress. Exercises in which the breath is held out are very powerful in their ability to help you work through deep-seated fears.

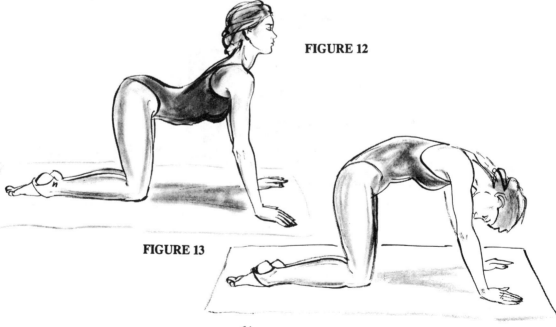

FIGURE 12

FIGURE 13

12. Extend your legs in front of you. Wrap the first two fingers of either hand around the corresponding big toe. As you inhale straighten up to whatever extent you can. As you exhale bring your nose towards your knees (figure 14). Continue at a good pace inhaling up and exhaling down.

Keep your diaphragm relaxed. Let your sacrum be a hinge. The *mantra* for this one is *Wha Guru* which means ecstasy beyond words or indescribable wisdom. As you inhale think *Wha* exhale think *Guru*. To end, assume the up position, exhale, hold the breath out as long as you comfortably can and apply Root Lock. Do this three times. Time open.

> *Relax like morning mist*
> *Kissed by the warmth*
> *Of the rising sun,*
> *Which is your spirit rising*
> *To be one with the One.*

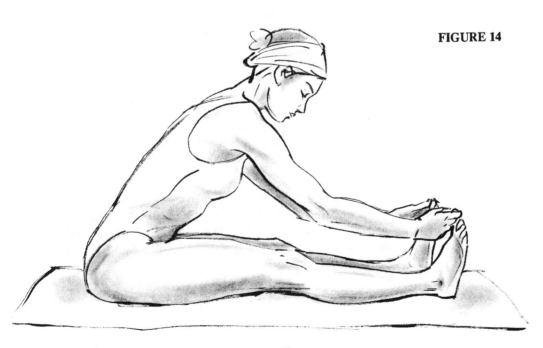

FIGURE 14

65

CHAPTER 6 - NAVEL POWER

In the yoga tradition the *Manipura Chakra* or Navel Center is considered to be a vortex of energy which corresponds to the area of the umbilicus or belly button. This center relates to will, patience, focus, and the ability to be unexploitable, and undefeatable.

Japanese martial arts traditions call this center is called the *hara*. It's said if this center is strong, no opponent can prevail against you.

In more practical terms, a strong Navel Center will give you the means to be very successful in life. In yoga, the Navel center has been linked to the element fire, which absorbs and purifies all obstacles. The Navel Center also relates to personal power. As previously stated, the Navel/Solar Plexus Center gathers, and consolidates energy, which in turn serves as fuel for the fire of our transformation.

In the womb we received nourishment through the navel via the umbilical cord. When that connection is severed at birth, the sustenance assumes a more subtle form. It's been said that the Divine Mother (energy of the universe) empowers us through the navel/solar plexus center. In other words when our Navel Center is consolidated, we can access a power source awesome in its magnitude.

There's a strong pulse beneath the navel. ideally this should be felt under the umbilicus. If this pulse is displaced, many chronic problems can ensue. A consistent yoga practice can usually alleviate this imbalance. If it persists consult a qualified health practitioner.

A strong Navel Center is considered to be a pre-requisite for the attainment of the long term benefits of Kundalini Yoga. It also gives you the discipline to stay one-pointed and do your practice every day. The following exercises will help strengthen your will, improve digestive functions, and strengthen and trim your abdomen.

1. Sit in a comfortable cross-legged position. Apply Neck Lock., the back of your tongue is pressing the roof of your mouth, and your eyes are 1/10 open looking down towards the tip of your nose (figure 1).

As you inhale contract the muscles of the rectum, sex organ, and navel point. In addition, pull your diaphragm up under the ribs. As you inhale feel that you're drawing energy into the body via the navel point. As you exhale relax the locks. Continue this breathing pattern for up to 3 minutes.

To end turn your eyes up towards the brow. Inhale, hold the breath and apply Root Lock. Hold the breath as long as you comfortably can. Now exhale, hold the breath out and apply *Maha Bhand* (contract the muscles of the rectum, sex organ, and navel point; in addition pull your diaphragm up under your ribs, and have your chin pulled back in neck lock). Inhale when you need to, relax the breath and meditate on the slow flow of the breath.

Again, have your eyes 1/10 open looking down towards the tip of the nose. Feel you have a sun in your belly. As you inhale feel the sun get hotter. As you exhale let it get brighter, as filaments of fire spread through your body to heal and energize you. Inhale *Sat* and exhale *Nam*. Continue in this way for as long as you'd like.

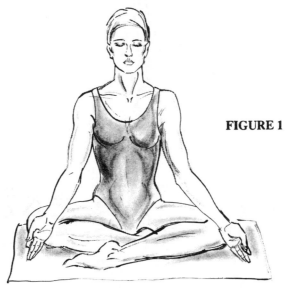

FIGURE 1

2. Lie on your back with your arms above your head on the floor. As you inhale raise the left straight up to 90 degrees. Exhale as you lower it. Then inhale as you raise your right leg, and exhale as you lower it (figure 2). Continue these alternate leg lifts for 3-5 minutes.

3. Immediately inhale and lift both legs to ninety degrees, and exhale as you lower them (figure 3). If your lower back feels put upon have your hands under the buttocks and bend your knees. Continue for 1-3 minutes.

4. Have your hands under the shoulders with your fingers pointing back towards the feet. Press yourself off the ground (figure 5) and do the Breath of Fire for 1-2 minutes. This one's called Wheel Pose. If you need to modify it press your hips up only and interlace your fingers under you.

Proceed immediately to the next exercise.

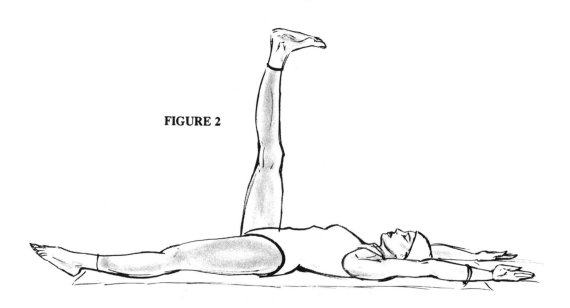

FIGURE 2

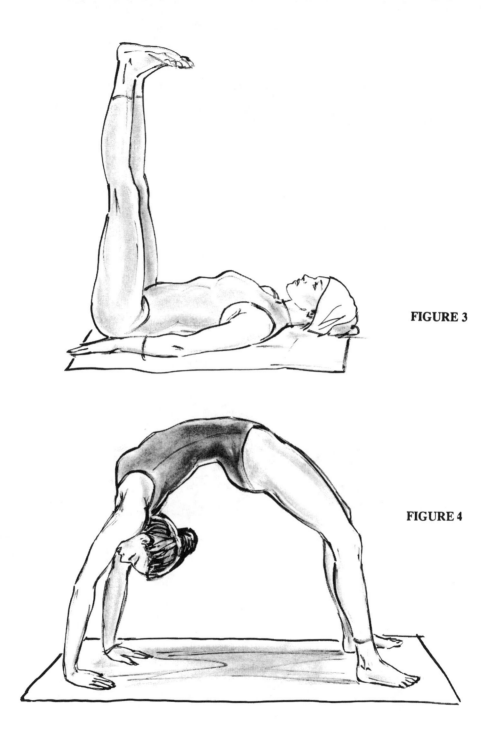

FIGURE 3

FIGURE 4

5. Stretch Pose. Lie on your back. Raise your head and heels 6 inches off the ground (figure 6). If your lower back feels put upon, to one leg at a time. Stare at your toes. Breath of Fire 1-2 minutes. Relax.

6. Wrap your arms around your bent knees and relax (figure 7). 1-3 minutes.

7. Inhale as you extend your legs to a 45 degree angle relative to the ground (figure 8). Exhale as you pull your knees into your chest (figure 7). Do this 3-5 minutes. You can increase the time to 15 min.

FIGURE 6

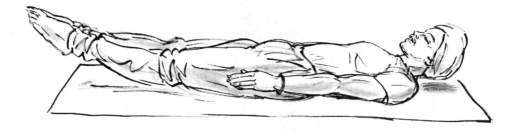

FIGURE 7

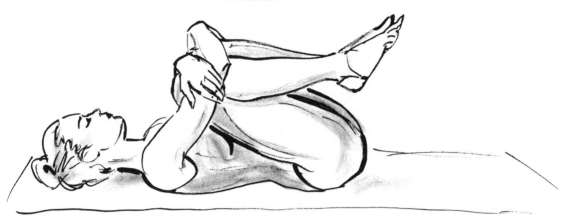

FIGURE 8

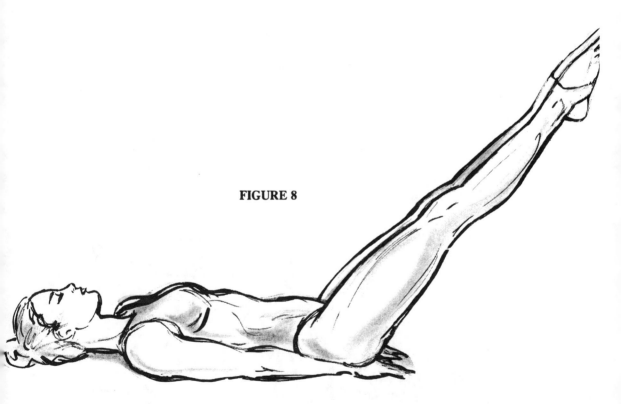

8. Still on your back, bend your left knee and pull it onto your chest. Begin rapid leg lifts with your right leg. Inhale to 90 degrees and exhale as you lower it to the floor (figure 9). Continue for 1 minute and switch sides. Continue for 1 minute more. Repeat this cycle 1 more time.

7. Stand with the upper arms hugging your ears, and your hands bent at the wrist with the palms facing the ceiling (figure 10). Inhale, and exhale as you bend from the waist and bring your hands to or towards the floor (figure 11). As you exhale squeeze Root Lock. Do this at a slow to a moderate pace for 2 minutes. Continue at an increased pace for 1 minute more.

Relax on your back.
Let your body find solace
In the floor's embrace.
Trade your tightness
For brightness,
Until no trace of stress remains.

FIGURE 9

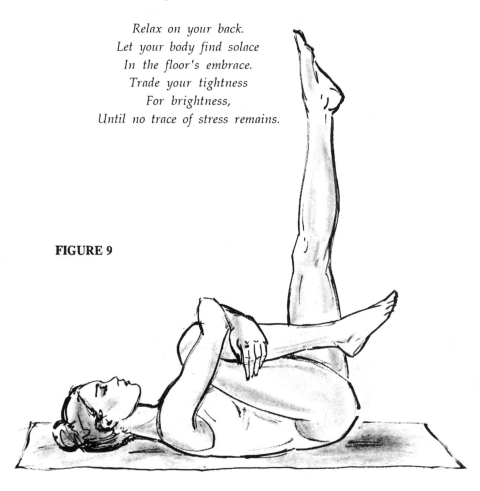

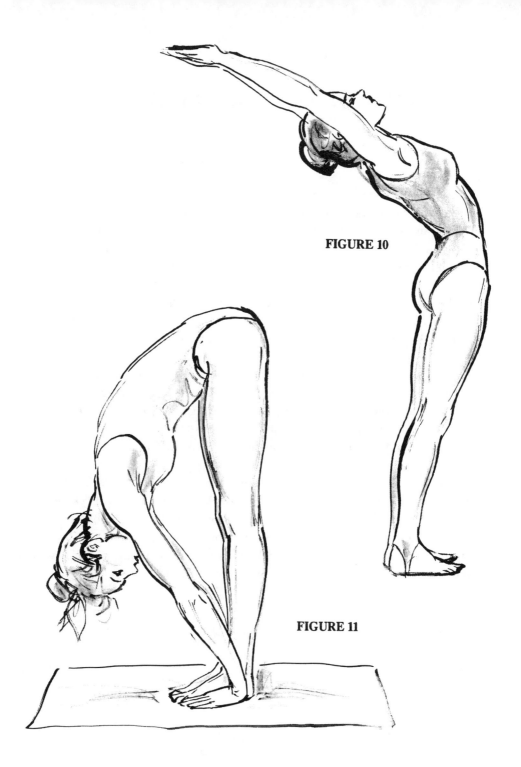

FIGURE 10

FIGURE 11

73

CHAPTER 7 - WARRIOR WORKOUT

"What doesn't kill you makes you strong."
- Nietzsche

In Kundalini Yoga we want to proceed with the realization that our true strength comes from within. We want to go beyond muscular strength alone, to faith in the flow of spirit. In light of this, breakthroughs become a way of life. Kundalini Yoga recognizes that a strong nervous system, and healthy glandular system, are pre-requisites for the Warriors' Way.

In the context of any exercise, when the going gets tough, remember these words. When your mind says, "No," let your spirit say,"Go" The moment we make a conscious decision to keep up, we become more than we were.

As a Teacher, I've seen that each exercise tends to elicit patterns of response similar to many life situations in which we're obliged to extend ourselves. If we can make keeping up a habit, then the next time we have a deadline to meet at work, or our softball team is playing for the championship, we'll have the confidence of knowing we have the resources to excel.

A Warrior is not necessarily a Conan-the-Barbarian type character hellbent on decimating the enemy, but someone who seeks to make a total investment in everything they do, for the sake of impeccability itself. He/she doesn't make value judgements on their actions, whether it be mowing the lawn or running a marathon. A Warrior seeks to balance celebration and discipline, and lives with a sense of calm urgency, keenly aware that life is a challenge and a gift.

Some people spend their whole lives waiting for, or resisting the tests they need to take. So, enter into the following sequence with firm resolve, grateful for the opportunity to work on yourself and grow.

This set is designed to help you eliminate toxins, improve circulation and give you aerobic benefits. It's important to realize that aerobic efficiency is your body's ability to utilize oxygen effectively, not the speed with which you can make your heart pound. So, get set to sweat, and go for the gold!

1. Standing. Have your arms at right angles, with the index fingers curled under the thumbs (figure 1). Run in place with the Breath of Fire. Knees high. Keep up! Although you're stationary you're actually going a long way. 5 minutes. Continue to the next exercise.

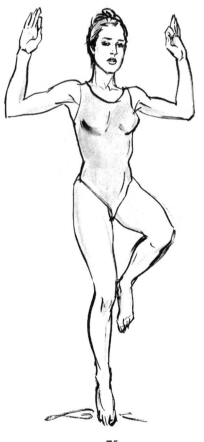

FIGURE 1

2. Assume Triangle Pose (figure 2), balancing equally on your feet and hands. The heels are off the ground. Inhale in Triangle Pose. Exhale as you press your heels to the floor.

Inhale. Exhale as you bend your elbows, and lower yourself so that your body is just off the ground, as if in a front push-up position (figure 3) .
Inhale. Exhale as you come into Cobra Pose (figure 4).
Inhale. Exhale as you return to Triangle Pose with your heels off the floor.

So, you inhale in each pose and exhale as you move to the next one. This is 1 cycle. Do this 26 of these 4 part cycles. Move immediately to the next exercise.

This exercise, called Sarbhang Dande Kriya puts a special pressure on your capillaries to help circulate the blood most effectively. Sikh warriors reportedly practiced this exercise 108 times 26 times a day. It's said that they developed the strength to hurl a spear through a steel shield.

FIGURE 2

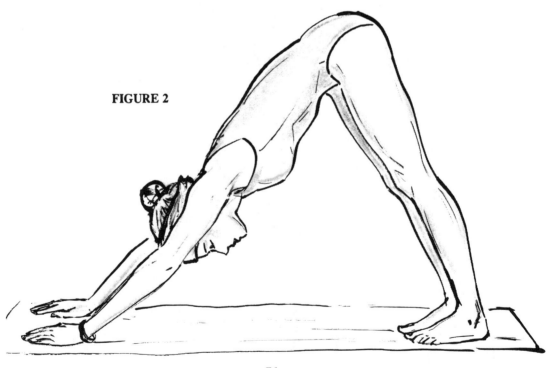

FIGURE 3

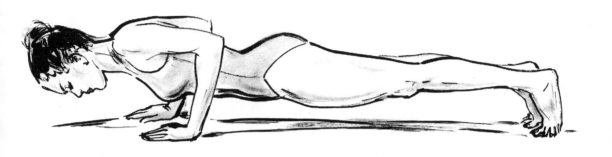

FIGURE 4

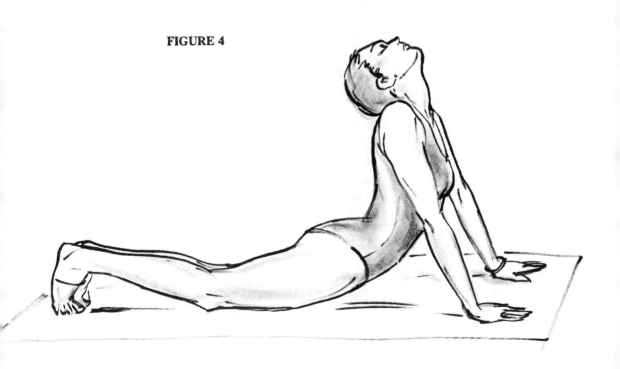

3. Sit in a cross-legged pose. Extend your left arm to the left parallel to the ground (figure 5), palm facing up. Breathe long and deeply through your nose for 2 minutes, then switch sides and continue for 2 more minutes .

Move immediately to the next exercise.

FIGURE 5

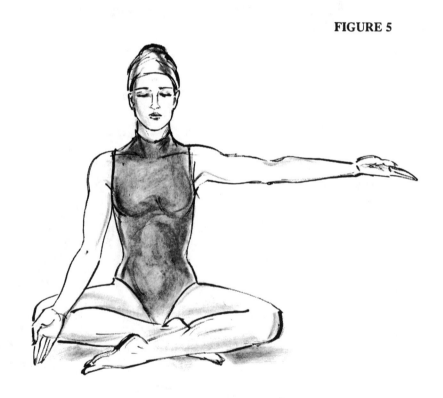

4. Have your legs in front of you wide. Hold onto the inside of your knees. (figure 6) Flex your spine in this pose. Inhale forward and exhale back. 1-3 minutes. Move to the next exercise.

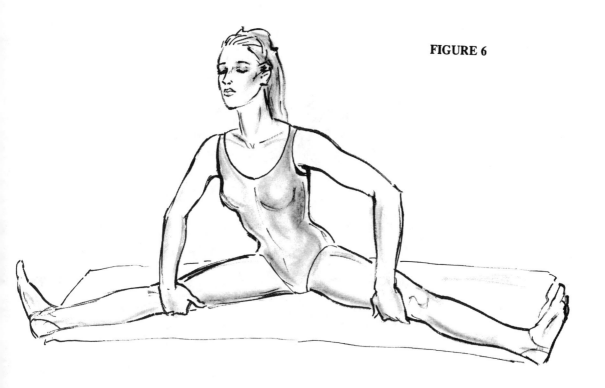

FIGURE 6

5. With your legs still wide, have your hands flat on the floor in front of you. Press. Try and lift yourself off the ground. 1-3 minutes. (figure 7) You should feel a pressure in the upper chest area. This one's for your lymphatic system. Proceed to the next one.

6. Enter into Frog Pose (figure 8).Your heels are together and off the ground. As you inhale straighten your knees and lower your head (figure 9). As you exhale return to the original position. Keep your elbows straight throughout the exercise. Do this 108 times! Proceed to the next one.

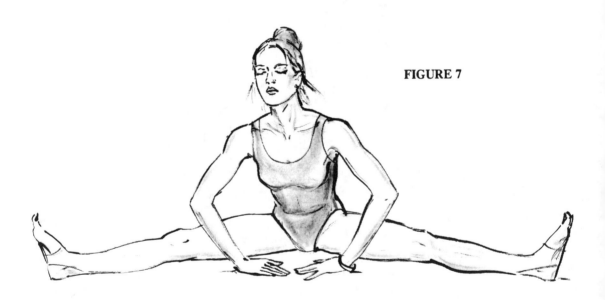

FIGURE 7

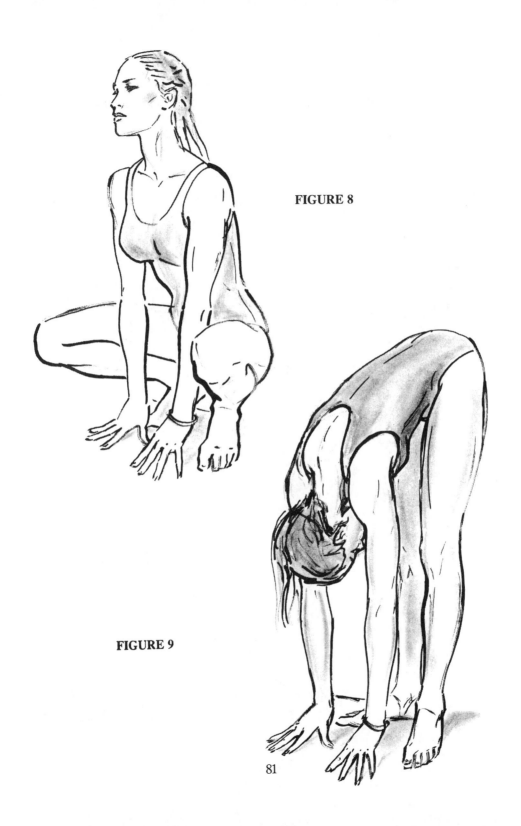

FIGURE 8

FIGURE 9

81

7. Sit on your heels in Rock Pose. As you inhale rise up off the heels, so that your body is perpendicular to the ground (figure 10). Press your hips forward somewhat. As you exhale return to the original position. Continue with vigor 108 times. Move to the next exercise.

8. Come into Triangle Pose (figure 11). Balance on your fingertips and toes (not shown). Breath of Fire 1-2 minutes. Go to the next exercise.

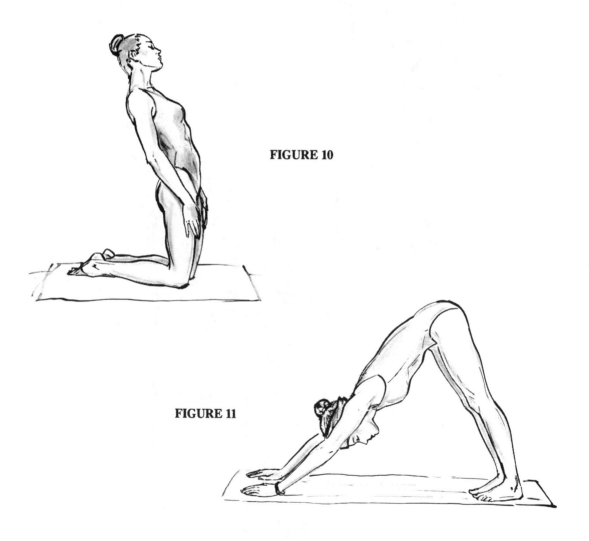

FIGURE 10

FIGURE 11

9. Lie on your stomach. Interlace your fingers at the small of the back. Raise your arms, upper body, and legs off the floor. (figure 12) Do Breath of Fire 2 minutes. Immediately move on.

FIGURE 12

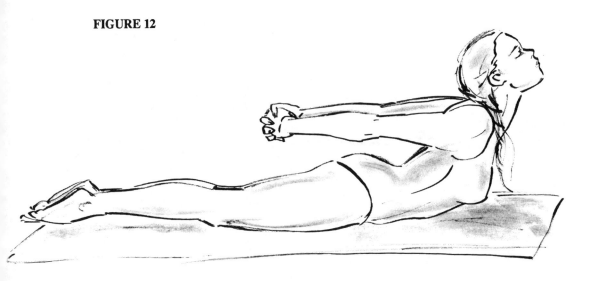

KEEP   UP!

10. Stay on your stomach. Your arms are by your sides palms facing down. As you inhale raise your hips off the ground. As you exhale lower them (figure 14). Again the movement is to the rhythm of the Breath of Fire. Continue for 2 minutes. Don't stop now. Move to the next one.

11. Still on your stomach, with your fingers interlaced, and arms pulled off your back (to give clearance to the heels). Kick your buttocks with alternate heels, exhaling every time you strike (figure 15). The breath is the Breath of Fire. The movement is rapid. Continue for 2 minutes. Move right along to the next one.

FIGURE 14

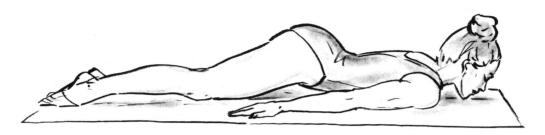

FIGURE 15

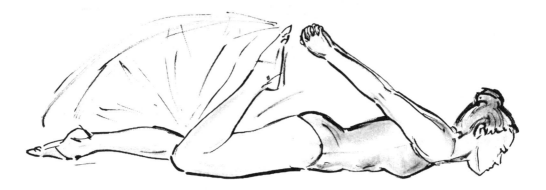

12. Lie on your stomach. Hold onto your right ankle with both hands. Extend your left leg straight and raise it off the ground. Rock on your stomach. Inhale back and exhale forward 1 minute. Switch sides, repeat. (figure 16)

Now hold both ankles and come up into Bow Pose. Rock on your stomach again. Inhale back and exhale forward 1 minute. (figure 17)

13 On your back again. As you inhale raise your legs straight up, and as you exhale lower them. Continue these double leg lifts for 2 minutes. If you need to, place your hands under your buttocks for support and/or bend your knees. Proceed to the next one.

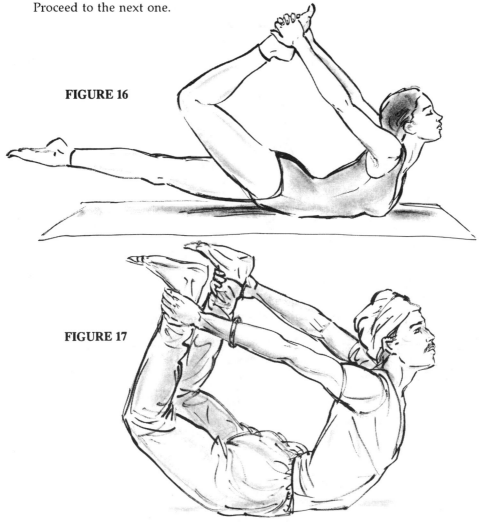

FIGURE 16

FIGURE 17

14 As you inhale raise the arms straight up to 90 degrees. Exhale raise your legs to 90 degrees. Inhale lower your legs, and exhale lower your arms (figure 18). Continue for one minute. Then do 30 seconds raising the right leg only, and thirty seconds raising the left leg only. With no break go to the next one .

15. From a cross-legged sitting position, without the help of your hands, stand up and press your hips forward (figure 19). Then sit down. Move quickly for 2 minutes. Forge ahead to the next exercise

FIGURE 18

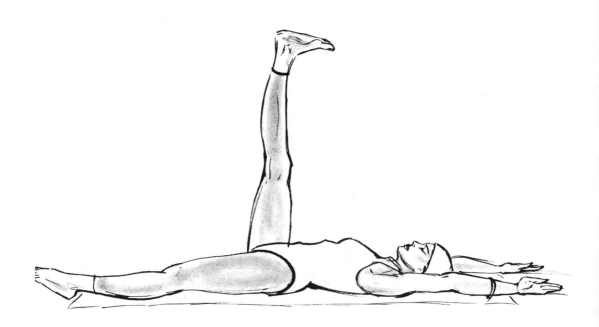

FIGURE 19

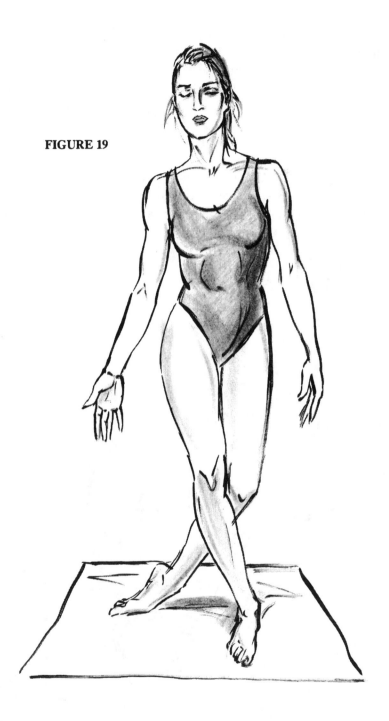

16. Sitting in easy pose. Interlace your fingers at the level of your diaphragm. Your arms are rounded. Twist with the Breath of Fire. Inhale as you pass center, and exhale to either extreme (figure 20). Continue for 2 minutes. Immediately do the next one.

17. Still in easy pose. Have your hands in fists at armpit level. Punch in concert with the Breath of Fire. Inhale as your fists pass each other and exhale to either extreme (figure 21). As one arms extends straight, the elbow of the opposite arm thrusts back past the plane of the body. Get furious. Smash your limitations to a pulp! Continue for 1-2 minutes. And finally move to the last exercise.

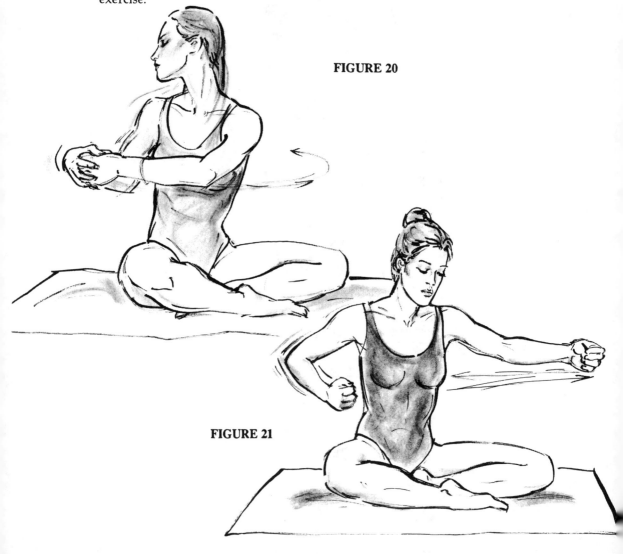

FIGURE 20

FIGURE 21

18 Sit on your heels in Rock Pose. Now all the toxins your surging bloodstream has delivered to your lungs are going to be expeditiously deported from your body

Your arms are straight with the palms down just above the knees. Open your eyes, incline your head slightly forward and stare at the floor. Stick your tongue out and do a powerful panting Breath of Fire (figure 22). 3 minutes.

> *Relax on your back,*
> *On a sea of Infinite calm.*
> *Having passed every test,*
> *Be healed, be balanced, be blessed.*

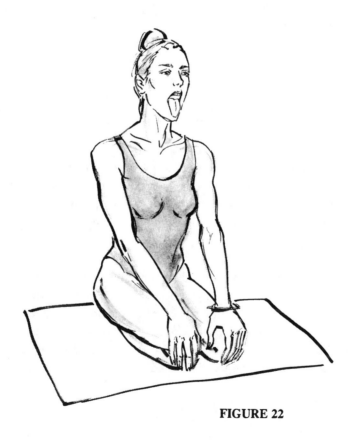

FIGURE 22

CHAPTER 8 - DIGESTIBLE YOU

There are no ironclad rules for a healthy digestive system. For every body type, constitution, and blend of environmental and genetic variables, there are as many appropriate considerations. Yoga advocates a vegetarian diet for health and moral reasons.

Most experts now agree that a person whose diet includes a large percentage of red meat and animal fat, runs a higher risk of a heart attack or cancer.

Also, meat and processed foods are difficult for your body to digest and eliminate. Over time they can create waste pockets, which get impacted in the folds of the intestines, and become a breeding ground for bacteria, and hinder your body's ability to extract nutritional value from food you eat.

Yoga as a way of life respects all life. It's obvious that no one can be perfect, but as conscious beings it's still incumbent on us to do the best we can. Yoga feels that killing animals to eat them is unnecessary and unhealthy. If you do decide to change your diet, do it gradually and consult a qualified health practitioner.

The quantity of food you eat is almost important as quality. Overeating can create an acid condition in the blood which makes you more susceptible to sickness. Yoga maintains that a nutritious and easily assimilated diet is best. A heavy diet puts undue strain on your system and siphons energy from the brain and higher centers.

To feel fresh when you get up (and do your yoga), I'd recommend that you not eat at least 3 hours before going to sleep. The old adage, "Eat to live; don't live to eat." is worth contemplating. Many of us use food to try and satisfy an ongoing emotional need. This creates a vicious cycle in which we overindulge because we're not happy with ourselves; then we're not happy with ourselves because we've overindulged!

We want to consciously use yoga to try and find a balance between extremes and make everything we do sacred. This means to try and have your meals in comfortable environments, and use food for its purpose intended: as fuel for the fire of our transformation.

The following exercises can be practiced as a set or individually. they will keep your digestive system running smoothly.

1. Sit with your legs crossed and hold your knees. Inhale through your mouth in successive sips. Take breaths in but don't let them out. Take about 16 of these sips. If you're not completely filled inhale (through your mouth) to your capacity and hold the breath.

Hold the breath, grind your stomach (figure 1). When halfway to the point where the breath cannot be held, put yourself in reverse and grind the other way. Exhale when you need to and repeat the entire exercise 1 more time.

If practiced twice daily on an empty stomach, this exercise can help you master your digestive system by adjusting the ileocecal valve and acid/alkaline balance in the stomach.

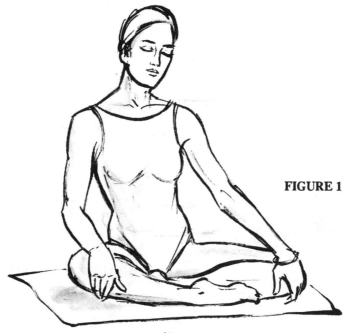

FIGURE 1

2. Lie on your back Have your arms by the sides palms facing down. If you need to put your hands under your buttocks for support. Inhale as you raise your legs to a 60 degrees angle (figure 2). Hold the breath for 10-15 seconds.

Exhale and bend your knees into the body (figure 3). Hold the breath out for 10-15 seconds.

Inhale and extend your legs to 60 degrees (figure 4). Hold the breath for 10 -15 seconds.

Exhale lower the legs to the floor, hold the breath out 10-15 seconds (figure 5).

Repeat this cycle 7 more times for a total of 8. As you hold the breath in and out mentally intone the *mantra Sa Ta Na Ma* in a consistent rhythm.

This one's called Pavan Sodhung Kriya Your liver will love you if you practice this. It's also extremely effective in helping to prevent constipation and other digestive dysfunctions. Ultimately this exercise can be practiced for up to 31 minutes! It's also a very effective technique for working through deep-seated fears. You may experience a slight sense of panic as you hold the breath out. Try to relax and let your fears evaporate.

FIGURE 2 , FIGURE 4

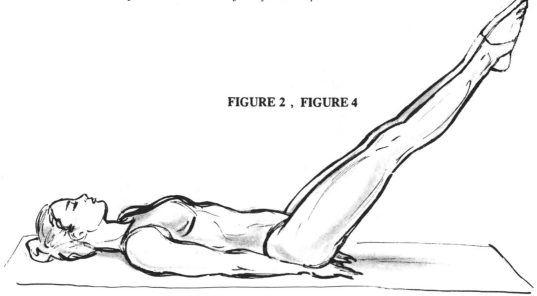

FIGURE 3

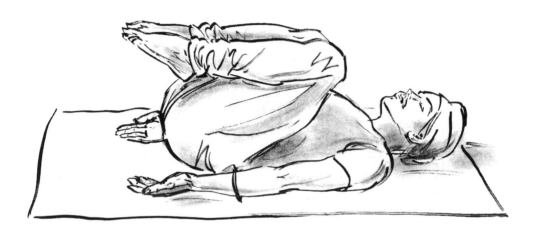

FIGURE 5

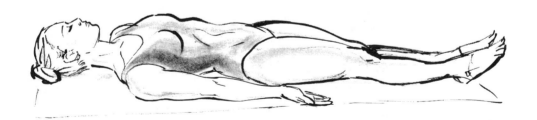

3. The following sequence is a powerful tonic for your digestive system.

A. Lie on your stomach. Your hands are in fists with the thumbs inside the fists. Place your hands under your hips, in the cavity where the thighs meet the body. Your face is facing forward, chin on the floor. Raise your legs up behind you and do Long Deep Breathing for 2 minutes. (figure 6)

FIGURE 6

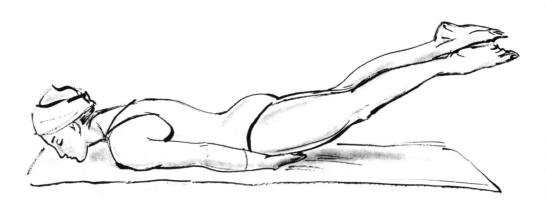

B. Sit on your heels. Press the fingertips and thumbtips of both hands into the navel. This *mudra* makes your hands into powerful focusers of energy (figure 7).

Lower your forehead to the floor. Again your fingertips are pressed deeply into the navel (figure 8). Breath of Fire 3 minutes.

Now, maintain the pose and inhale through your nose and exhale through the teeth, making a hissing sound. Continue this breath for 3-5 minutes.

And last but not least, breathe long and deeply through your nose for at least 3 more minutes (you can do this longer if you'd like).

FIGURE 8

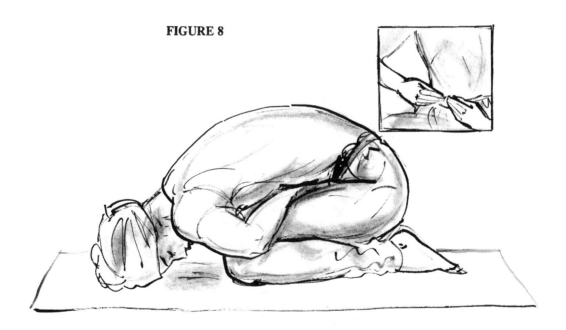

C. Remain on your heels and sit up. Extend your arms up so that the upper arms are hugging your ears. Interlace your fingers so that your index fingers are extended .

This is *Sat Kriya*. Say *Sat* as you pull your navel in. Say *Nam* as you relax your navel (figure 10). Bring your mind to this exercise. Feel *Sat* at your navel, and *Nam* rising up your spine. Continue for at least 3 minutes. To end inhale hold the breath and apply Root Lock. Then exhale hold the breath out and squeeze up again. Relax.

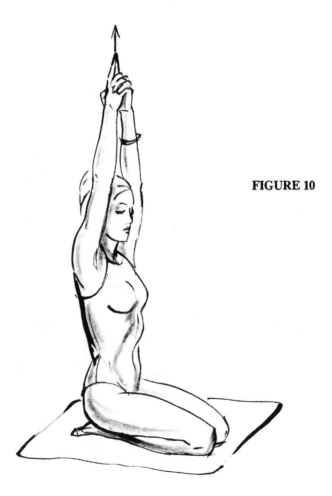

FIGURE 10

CHAPTER 9 - WHAT TO DO
FOR THE SUGAR BLUES

Chronic symptoms, which include late afternoon low periods, high and low mood swings, compulsive eating patterns, and fatigue, are common modern day complaints. These symptoms are now being linked to hypoglycemia, Candida (yeast intolerance), and other organic imbalances.

Proper diet is intrinsic to overcoming these. Dietary considerations, notably the elimination of sugar, frequently play a key role in achieving a state of homeostasis in your life.

In yoga we seek to take responsibility for every area of our lives. So, read labels, consult a good nutritionist, and above all, tune into your body and its signals.

It's easy to rationalize about the typical American diet with, "Everyone else seems to get away with it, why can't I?" The fact is that no one "gets away" with anything. In our culture old age has become synonomous with senility and an alarming incidence of cancer and heart disease. Now's the time to take matters into your own hands, and create the habits and perspective which will save you from suffering needlessly.

Our approach in the following sequence is to strengthen the immune system, revitalize the organs, and bring balance to the body's metabolic functions.

1. The following breathing exercise will be helpful when the late afternoon lows create a dip in your day.

Sitting Straight: have your elbows against the sides, forearms angled at a 45 degree angle. Inhale in 8 parts through your nose, then exhale in 1 part. Your palms are facing up with the index fingers curled under the thumb. Your eyes are 1/10 open looking down towards the tip of the nose. 3-11 minutes.

2. Sit on your heels. Extend your arms straight up so that the upper arms are hugging the ears. The heels of the hands are meeting with the fingers angling away from the base of the hands at an angle of 45 degrees (figure 1).

As you inhale raise your body off the heels 3/4 of the way to perpendicular. As, you rise up press your hips forward and arms back. Exhale and return to your heels. Do this one slowly and breathe deeply.

Practice this up to 11 minutes, although you may want to start with 1-3 minutes, and build up the time over time.

This exercise, if practiced on a regular basis will help you attain and maintain the glow of youth. It works on the adrenals, thyroid, and thymus glands, as well as the pancreas, and liver, organs stressed by hypoglycemia and related imbalances.

3. Sit with your legs crossed and again extend your arms straight up. The palms are pressed together. As you inhale twist left. As you exhale twist right (figure 2). 1-3 minutes with a powerful breath. To end inhale center. Stretch up.

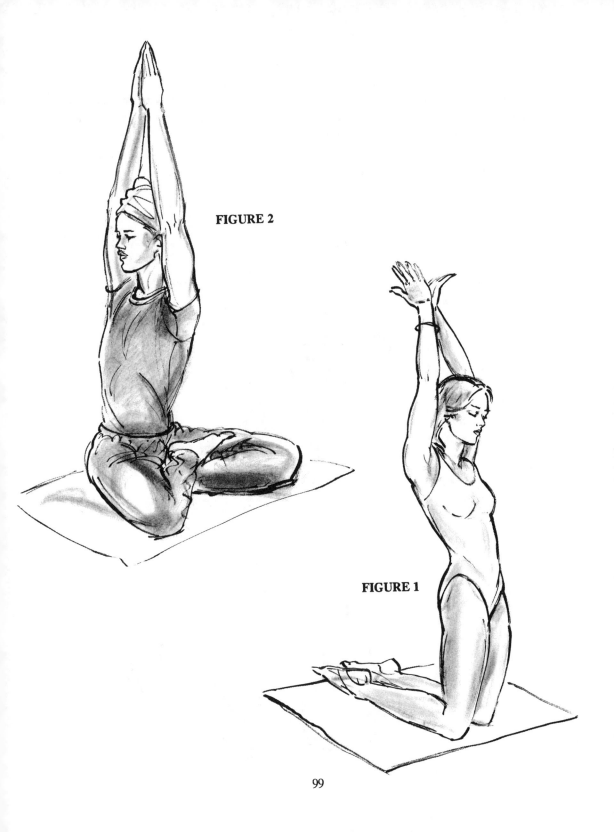

FIGURE 2

FIGURE 1

99

3. Still sitting with your legs crossed. Interlace your fingers with the palms facing away from you at the level of the hairline. The elbows are bent. Inhale pull your hands back and press your face forward (figure 3). Exhale return to the original position. Continue at a moderate pace 3 minutes. This one can ultimately be done for 11 minutes.

Relax on your back.
Tax yourself no more
Rather receive a refund
From the Government of Grace.

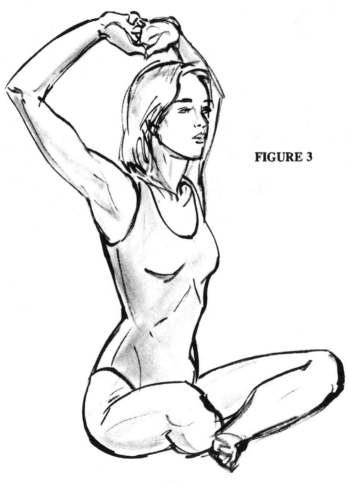

FIGURE 3

CHAPTER 10 - HAVE A HEART

The heart is a marvelous mechanism which keeps time with our lives. It's never had a day off! In spite of its perpetual motion, it needs to be exercised as any other muscle does. In addition, a proper diet is intrinsic to the health of the heart.

The following exercises will strengthen your heart and work on the Heart Center, which relates to the human attributes of love, compassion, and spirit Those whose heart centers have blossomed are considered to be humanly human, and Divinely inspired.

1. Sitting with a straight spine. Extend your arms to 60 degrees with the hands bent at the wrists and the palms facing the ceiling (figure 1). Long Deep Breathing. 1-3 minutes.

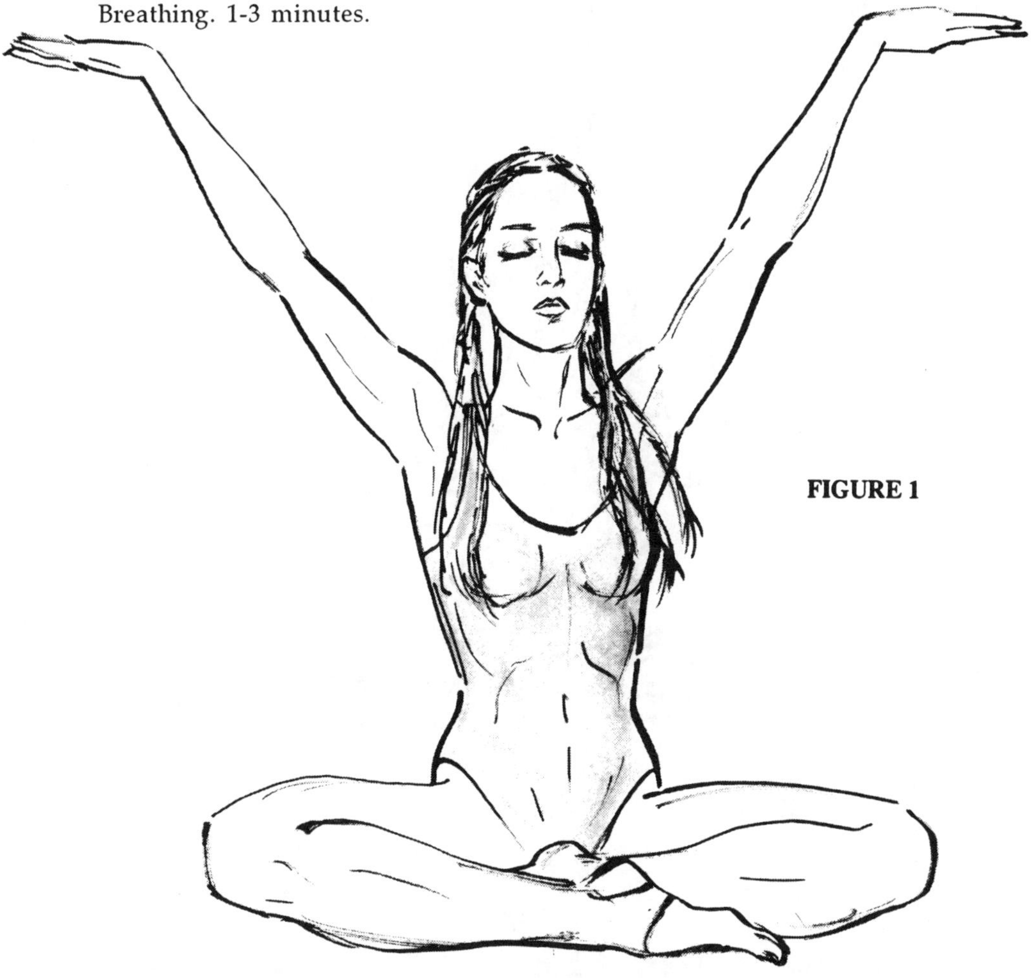

FIGURE 1

As you inhale, feel that the light of the breath is streaming in through the center of the palms, down the arms to the sternum. As you exhale feel this light at the sternum expand to fill body. Continue 1-3 minutes.

Bring your hands into Prayer Pose. Do Breath of Fire 1-3 minutes (figure 2,)

Inhale, hold the breath, apply *Maha Bhand* pressing your hands together hard.

Repeat with the breath held out. Inhale, relax the breath and meditate.

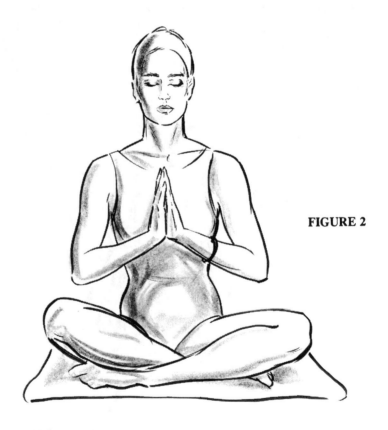

FIGURE 2

2. Frog Pose: Heels together, knees bent, your arms are between your knees, elbows straight. Your fingertips are on the floor. As you inhale straighten your knees and lower your head (figure 3), as you exhale return to the original position (figure 4). Continue at a good pace 26-40 times.

Now inhale into the up position (figure 3), maintain the pose and exhale With the breath held out pump your stomach as long as you can. Inhale when you must and continue to pump your stomach with the breath held out. Do this up to 8 times.

Flatten your feet and let yourself hang over, like a rag doll.

FIGURE 3   **FIGURE 4**

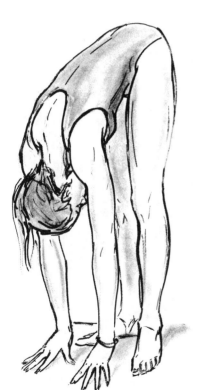

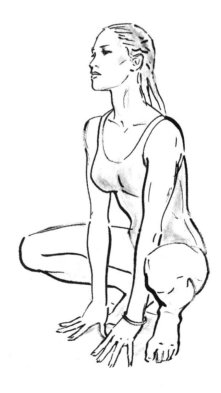

3. Slowly stand up. Interlace your fingers at the small of the back. As you inhale raise your arms up off the back, simultaneously raising one knee (figure 5). Exhale as you lower the legs and arms. Alternate legs. 3 minutes and immediately move to the next exercise.

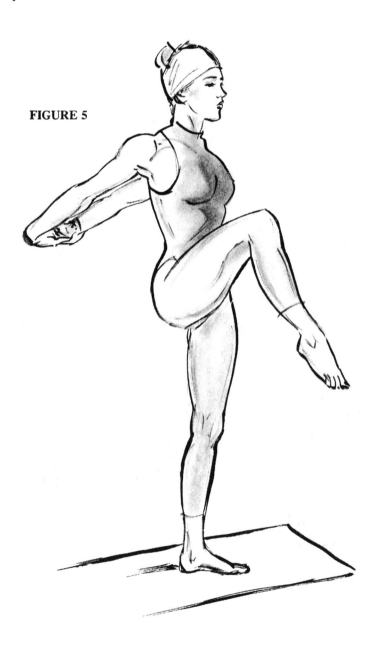

FIGURE 5

4. Still standing. Come up on your toes. Your arms are stretched up with the fingers wide (figure 6). Breath of Fire 2 minutes. Your circulatory system will love you for this! Relax on your back.

5. Elbow Platform Pose: Balance on your elbows and heels only, head back. Breath of Fire 1-2 minutes. Relax.

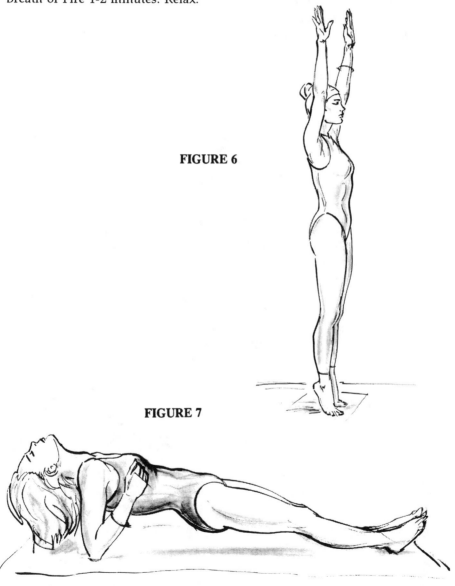

FIGURE 6

FIGURE 7

105

6. Sit with a straight spine. Press the palms of the hands together so that the fingertips are at brow level (figure 8). Your hands are 3 inches in front of your face. Hold this pose. Let the breath regulate itself. Do this for 11 minutes. To end, interlace your fingers, inhale, and stretch up. Really stretch.

According to yoga, this exercise, called Jot Kriya, can help prevent or cure heart problems. Heart patients, after checking with their physicians, should practice this exercise for 1-2 minutes and slowly build up the time.

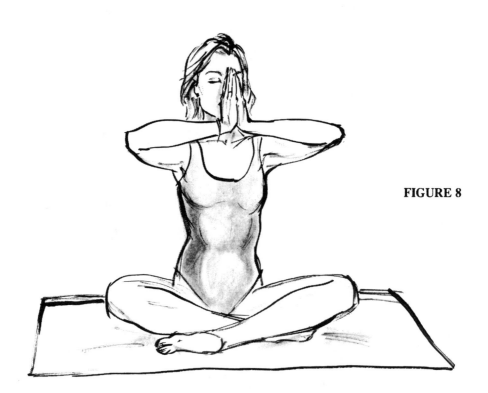

FIGURE 8

CHAPTER 11 - BRIGHT AND BEAUTIFUL

The exercises in this chapter will help you increase your charisma, radiance, projection, and luck, by strengthening your aura, or magnetic field.

According to the science of yoga, a strong magnetic field will give you the ability to compute, through the force of your radiance, beyond time and space, transform your environments, and heal, uplift, and inspire, everyone in your sphere.

1. A. Triangle Pose. Make your body into a triangle by balancing your weight equally on your feet and hands. Raise your left leg as high as you can (figure 1). Inhale, and exhale as you bend your elbows and lower your hair-line towards the ground. Do 26-40 of these Triangle Pose Push-ups. Meditate for a minute and switch sides.

FIGURE 1

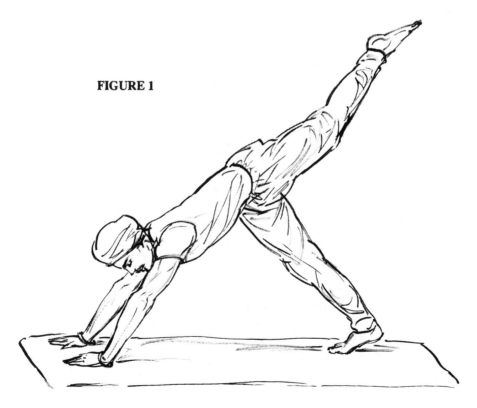

B Sit with your legs crossed. Extend your left arm straight out from the shoulder with the fingers of the left hand pointing left, so that the left palm faces forward. Have the right arm extended straight in front of you palm down. Move the right hand under the left wrist, and hold the left hand from over the top. Pull back on the fingers.

As you inhale raise the arms to 60 degrees (figure 2). As you exhale lower them just above the shins. Keep your elbows straight throughout. Breathe and move powerfully for 5 minutes, then meditate and consolidate your gains.

C. Sitting with your legs crossed. Inhale as you swing your arms back behind you (figure 3). Exhale and swing your arms forward so that your hands come up to eye level (figure 4). 5 minutes. As your hands come up to eye level, blink your eyes open. As your arms go back close your eyes. Feel your energy field.

FIGURE 2

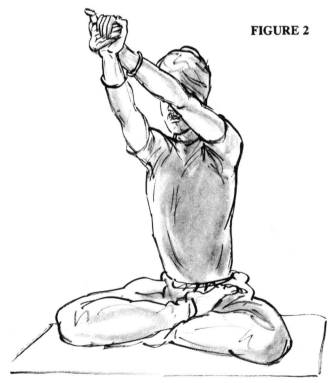

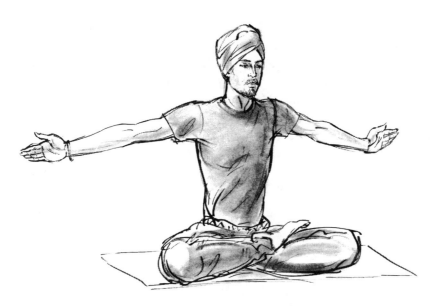

FIGURE 3

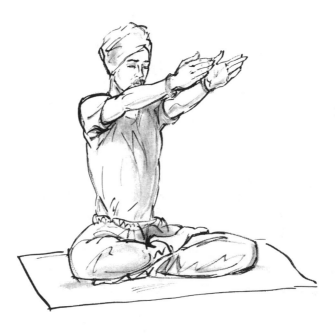

FIGURE 4

109

D. Upon completing the exercise, meditate for 1-2 minutes. Then, with the elbows bent, have your hands about 6-8 inches apart at the level of the sternum. Gaze at the space between the hands (figure 4). Try and discern the energy field between your hands. It may appear like fine smoke or glitter.

Close your eyes. Your hands are still in front of your sternum. Slowly move your hands towards one another, almost touching, then away. As the hands get closer you will probably feel the magnetic field between them get more dense, and as they separate you'll feel it expand.

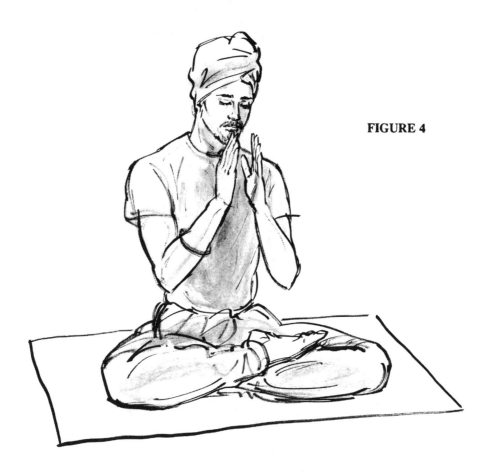

FIGURE 4

2. *The following sequence is called Ego-Eradicator. Semantically speaking, we don't really want to diminish our ego in yoga, we want to expand it to include greater possibilities. When we increase our radiance, or sphere of influence, we expand our horizons and exert a positive influence wherever we go.*

A   Sit between your heels. If this is not possible for you sit on your heels or with your legs crossed. Now raise your arms to a 60 degree angle with your elbows straight. Your fingertips are curled in, pressing against the mounds at the base of the fingers. Your thumbs are pointing straight up (figure 5). This is called Eagle Pose. Breath of Fire. 3 minutes

Visualize and feel a rainbow of light between your thumbs, pulsating and brightening as you breathe. After 3 minutes inhale, hold the breath and slowly bring your thumbs towards one another like two powerful magnets, attracting and repelling at the same time, the energy intensifying between them. When you cannot hold the breath any longer, let your thumbtips meet (without looking up), and relax the breath as you let the thumbs come apart and the arms float down to the sides as if through water.

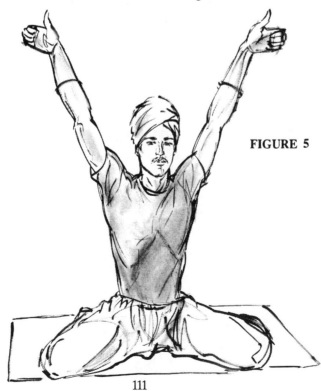

FIGURE 5

111

B. Remaining between your heels, place your hands on your shoulders, fingers in front, thumbs in back. As you inhale extend the arms up and out to sixty degrees. Exhale as you bring your hands back to your shoulders. Continue hard and fast for 3 minutes. Then inhale hold the breath and apply Root Lock, then hold the breath out and apply *Maha Bhand*. Inhale, relax the breath and meditate.

C. Still between your heels. With your hands on your shoulders, fingers in front thumbs in back, do Breath of Fire for 3 more minutes. To end hold the breath in and then out for as long as you comfortably can, with the locks applied.

Our Radiance-
Cloak of Consciousness,
Perfume of Prayer-
We bring hope everywhere,
And fling healing like luminous confetti
At the parade of all souls.

We are Viceroys of the King,
And carry His Great Light through the world,
And let Truth be shown,
The wings of Majesty unfurled.

--Ravi Singh

CHAPTER 12 - PICK ME UP EXERCISES

These exercises represent a real alternative to any kind of artificial stimulants. Coffee, cigarettes, sugar, and various kinds of drugs may seem to work temporarily, but in the long run they take their toll on your body. Conscious breathing gives you pure energy. It leaves no toxic residue and helps you eliminate the impurities of the past.

When you come home after work feeling tired and testy, instead of slumping down in front of the tv, do some yoga. Thus you become your own energy source. In light of our Kundalini Yoga practice, we want to establish a habit of hardiness, a willingness to go that extra mile, to be able to meet our responsibilities with integrity, and give joyful expression to our indefatigable spirit.

1. Have your hands in prayer pose. Focus at the brow and inhale in four equal parts and exhale in four equal parts. (figure 1). Continue this segmented breathing for 3-5 minutes.

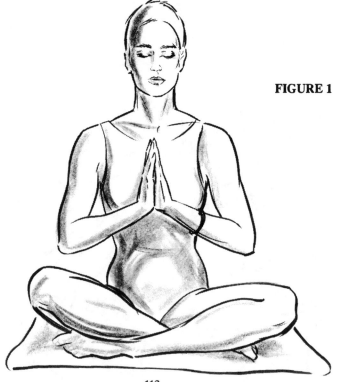

FIGURE 1

2. Yoga Push-ups. Assume the standard push-up position with the tops of the feet on the ground. The toes are not curled under. Inhale. Exhale as you bend your elbows and lower your body just off the ground. Continue with a powerful breath 26 times (figure 2).

3. Lie on your stomach. Grab your ankles and rise up into Bow Pose (figure 3). Breath of Fire 1-2 minutes.

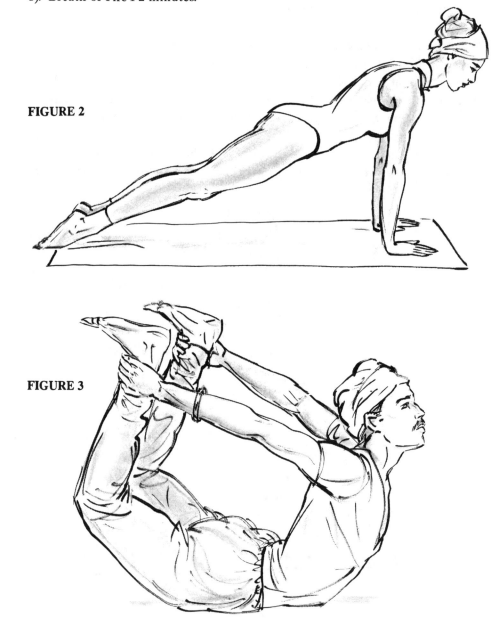

FIGURE 2

FIGURE 3

4. Have your hands in fists with the thumbs inside the fists, under the hips where the thighs meet the body. Your face is facing forward with your chin on the ground. Inhale as your raise your left leg. Exhale as you raise your right leg simultaneously lowering the left (figure 4). The legs will pass one another in mid-air. Continue for 2 minutes.

5. Still on your stomach. Have your hands under the shoulders palms down. Raise your head and upper body into Cobra Pose (figure 5) Breath of Fire 1 minute, then apply Root Lock with the breath held and expelled.

Now maintaining Cobra Pose, have your legs wide. Inhale as you look to your right foot, and exhale as you look at your left foot. Do this 5 times then slowly ease out of the pose.

FIGURE 4

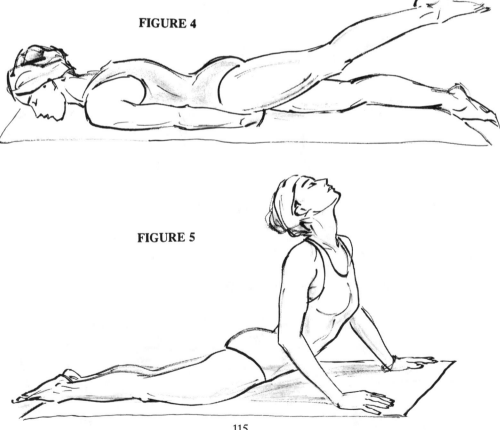

FIGURE 5

6. Hold opposite wrists behind your back. Rock gently on your stomach from side to side.

7. With your arms by your sides, imagine you're a bundle of logs. Without using your arms, roll over a few times in one direction, then the other. Continue this Bundle Roll for at least 2 minutes. Relax on your back

9. For energy anytime: Sit with your legs crossed, and block your left nostril with your left thumb. The fingers of the left hand are pointing straight up (figure 6). Do Breath of Fire through the right nostril for 3 minutes.

FIGURE 6

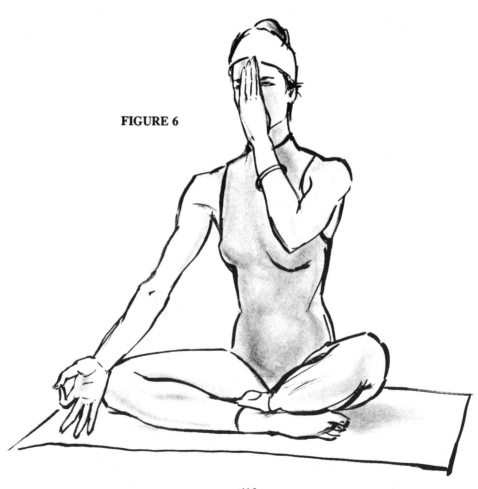

CHAPTER 13 - WHEN STRESS GETS THE BEST OF YOU WHAT TO DO

Stress is a broad term which includes any invasive influence on our well being. Stress can be nutritional, physical, psychological, emotional, and environmental. Each of these tends to make us more susceptible to the influences of the others. Consequently, what most of us experience as stress, to varying degrees, is a combination of all of these.

Outside influences known as stressors trigger extreme responses in our bodies. Over time our internal systems get worn down and we begin to exhibit any number of symptoms.These are signals from our body/mind apprising us of an imbalance vying for resolution. When we ignore these signals, and fail to make the necessary lifestyle adjustments, serious health problems often ensue.

One would have to live in a vacuum to avoid stress completely (and I'm not even sure this would work!). The bottom line, I feel, in the quest to make stress less, is to strike a perspective, which makes adversity adventure, and life's challenges a test to grow by.

The following sequence will strengthen your nerves. In addition I have included a breath meditation to help you recover from the effects of long term stress, as well as a meditation for tranquility.

Kundalini Yoga is yoga of nerve strength. Daily practice will make you strong as steel and steady as stone.

Before you begin this sequence, make sure you're properly warmed up.

1. Standing. Your legs are as wide as possible, with the feet flat and toes pointing forward. If you can, grasp your big toes. If this isn't possible, you can have your hands flat on the floor. Raise your head and arch your spine. Grip the ground with your feet. Long Deep Breathing 1-3 minutes (figure 1).

2. Lie on your stomach. Come up on your elbows with the hands in fists at shoulder level. Now curl your toes under and raise your body off the ground Then raise your right leg off the floor (figure 2). Long Deep Breathing 1-2 minutes. Switch sides. Relax.

3. Sit on your heels. Extend your arms straight out to the sides, palms facing out and fingers pointing up. Breathe long and deeply for 1-3 minutes then do Breath of Fire for 1-3 minutes (figure 3). Relax.

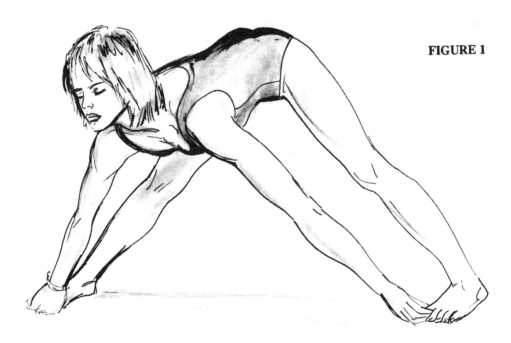

FIGURE 1

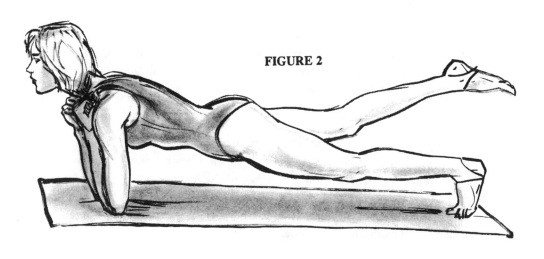

FIGURE 2

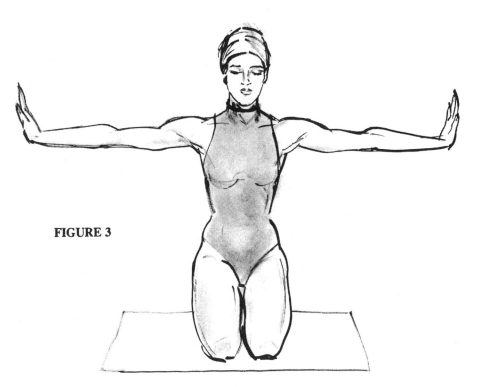

FIGURE 3

119

4. Come into a front push-up position with the tops of the feet on the ground. Your head is up, with your eyes open staring straight ahead (figure 4) Do Long Deep Breathing 1-3 minutes, then Breath of Fire for 1-3 minutes more.

5. Back Platform Pose. With your legs extended in front of you, support yourself with your hands. Raise yourself off the ground with your head back (figure 5). Do Long Deep Breathing 1-3 minutes, then Breath of Fire 1-3 minutes more. Relax.

6. Sit with your legs crossed. Extend your arms straight in front of you at shoulder level. Your left hand is in a fist with the thumb pointing up. Wrap the left hand around the right fist. The sides of the thumbs are together. Stare at your thumbnails (figure 6). Inhale for 5 seconds, exhale for 5 seconds, and hold the breath out for 15 seconds or more. Begin with 3-5 minutes of practice and build up to 11 minutes over time.

FIGURE 4

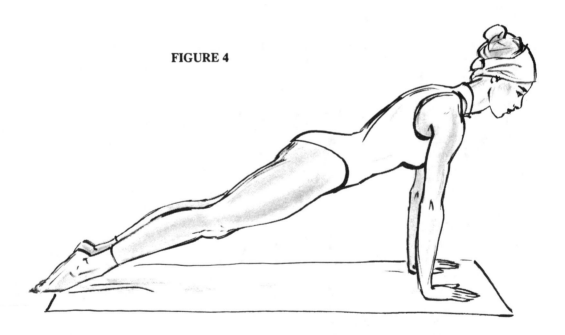

FIGURE 5

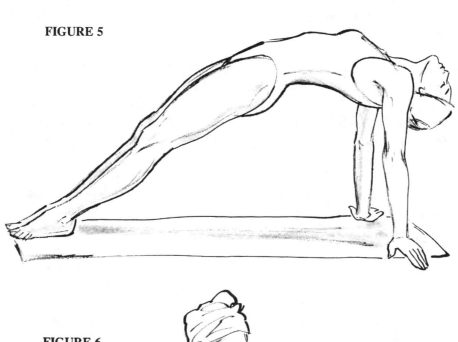

FIGURE 6

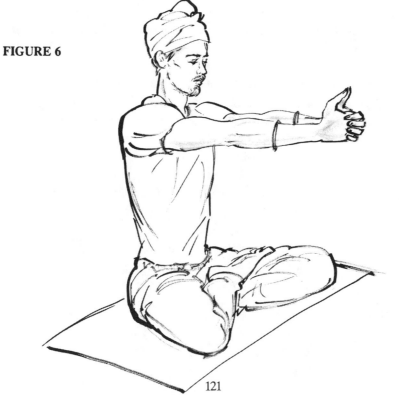

121

7. And this is called Meditation to Tranquilize Your Mind. Sit in a comfortable pose. Have your elbows bent, with your forearms parallel to the ground. The hands are at sternum level.

Bend the index finger of each hand in towards the palm. The index fingers are pressed together along the second joint. The middle fingers are extended and meet fingerprint to fingerprint. The thumbs also meet fingerprint to fingerprint, and are pointing straight back towards the sternum. The ring and little fingers are curled in towards the palm (figure 7). Hold this configuration about 4 inches in front of the body.

Inhale and hold the breath. Mentally repeat *Sat Nam* 11 to 21 times. Exhale hold the breath out and repeat *Sat Nam* mentally for an equal duration. Do this for 3 minutes any time you'd like a little tranquility in your life.

True wisdom belongs to anyone who understands that the mind by its very nature is dual. For every yes, a no is lurking somewhere near, and vice versa. Without the focus that conscious work on oneself engenders, we find ourselves slaves to the mind's meanderings, unable to commit, concentrate, manifest, or intuit.

The yogic or meditative mind finds ecstasy in neutrality. In light of this one sees pain/pleasure, gain/loss, love/hate, and even life/death, as two sides of the same coin. When this state of mind has been attained one is truly free.

You've attained
The sacred summit,
Above the hurry and worry of the world.
Let the flag of your higher self
Be unfurled
In the wind of the breath,
And hold dominion over a Destiny.

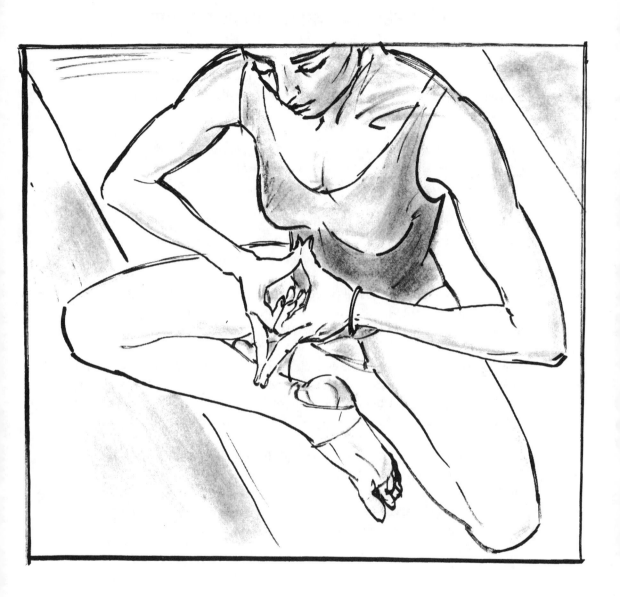

CHAPTER 14 - BEST BEFORE BED

A healthy sleep life depends on the following things: A strong and balanced nervous system, a healthy glandular system, and attitudes, environments, and lifestyle considerations conducive to relaxation.

Our bodies are tuned to a circadian rhythm. This means that our systems respond to the timetable of the sun. Yoga maintains that it's best to get up before the sun rises, and go to sleep early enough to make this feasible.

If you adhere to the appropriate lifestyle considerations you'll find that 6 hours of sleep is more than enough for you. Ultimately you'll find that 8 hours of sleep will prove to be more enervating than restful.

A cardinal rule for successful sleep is DON'T EAT AT LEAST 3 HOURS BEFORE GOING TO SLEEP. Going to sleep on a full stomach puts stress on the very systems which need to regenerate.

Many episodes of insomnia or lethargy stem from energy imbalances, and unresolved emotional issues and anxiety. Meditating before bed on a regular basis can help you put the day behind you and give you the organizational and intuitive capacity to make the most of the day ahead.

In yogic terminology, true sleep, deep and dreamless, is called the *turya* state, known as The Sleep of the Saints. The R.E.M. (rapid eye movement) phase of sleep is essentially your subconscious trying to clear itself. This tends to be stressful to your nervous system, disturbing dreams especially. Meditation filters subconscious stress in a more effective and enduring way

The following techniques work on your nervous system, energy and glandular balance, the digestive system, and deep relaxation.

The first exercise, although basic, is a very effective pre-bed technique. Do it honestly and you'll be able to get up on a dime, whatever time you program yourself to awaken.

When we work on the sciatic nerve (the longest nerve in the nervous system), we bring balance to our emotions, digestive and nervous systems.

1. Sitting, extend your legs in front of you. Reach down and pull back on your toes, if this isn't possible hold onto your ankles or calves. Stretch down (figure 1) and breathe long and deeply through your nose.

You can do the following visualization to enhance the exercise. Feel you're inhaling through the heels up the backs of the legs to the tailbone, exhale up the spine like a white wave. Let it crest over your crown. Focus at the brow, and of course, inhale think *Sat* and exhale think *Nam* . Time open.

To end inhale, exhale and stretch, applying *Mul Bhand*. Do this as many times as you'd like.

FIGURE 1

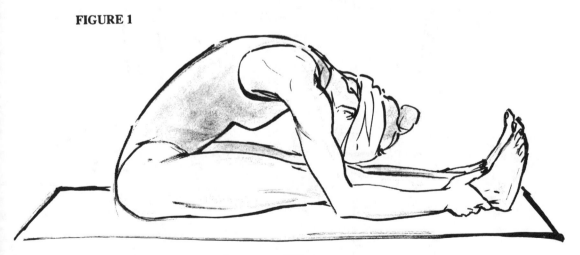

2. The next exercise, done before bed, will help your nerves to relax. It also will reverse the flow of cerebral-spinal fluid, so that the day's momentum can become sleep's benign inertia. It's called Bridge Pose.

With your feet flat and knees bent, press your hips up, with your elbows straight, and head back (figure 2). Hold the pose and squeeze *Mul Bhand* for 1-3 minutes with a normal breath, then do Long Deep Breathing for 1-3 minutes more. Relax.

FIGURE 2

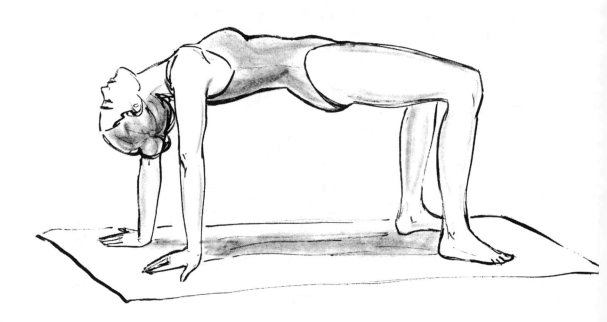

3 Lie on your back. Have the arms straight up from the shoulders, perpendicular to the ground, palms facing in towards one another. Take a few deep breaths. Now inhale hold the breath, make your hands into tight fists, and pull your fists toward the sternum. The elbows bend outwards (figure 3) Get as angry as you can. Pull! When you can't hold the breath any more, let the hands come to the sternum as you exhale. Repeat the exercise one more time.

FIGURE 3

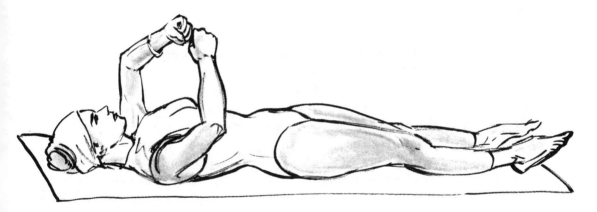

4. This one's called *Shabd Kriya*:

Sit in a comfortable position with your spine straight. Your hands are in your lap with your right hand over the left (figure 4). The thumbtips are pressed together and pointing forward. Your eyes are 1/10 open, looking down towards the tip of the nose.

Inhale in 4 equal parts through the nose so that by the 4th inhale your lungs are filled. As you inhale in 4 parts, mentally intone *Sa Ta Na Ma* (Existence, Life, Death, Rebirth).

Hold the breath and mentally repeat *Sa Ta Na Ma* 4 times for a total of 16 beats.

Now exhale in two equal parts mentally repeating *Wahay Guru*, Indescribable Wisdom, or Ecstasy Beyond Words.

Do this at a slow pace for 11 to 62 minutes.

To reiterate: You inhale in 4 parts, hold for 16 counts, and exhale in 2 breaths thinking *Sa Ta Na Ma* and then *Wahay Guru*

Shabd Kriya can help you regenerate the nervous system. This is important for those who have a history of drug abuse, coffee consumption, and long term stress.

This before-bed meditation will give you the power of rhythmic existence, so that your timing, temperament, and temerity, will help you glide through life's travails. It will help you compete, create, and relate with power and grace.

Shabd Kriya is also a very effective measure against jet-lag and the overall stress which travelling imposes. It helps your nervous system and magnetic field to adjust when you're thrust out of your normal frame of reference.

It's recommended you do this for at least 31 minutes after flying, and for at least 11 minutes after having taken a long car or train trip.

Shabd Kriya will help you sleep deep and wake up feeling like a million. Make it a nightly ritual.

128

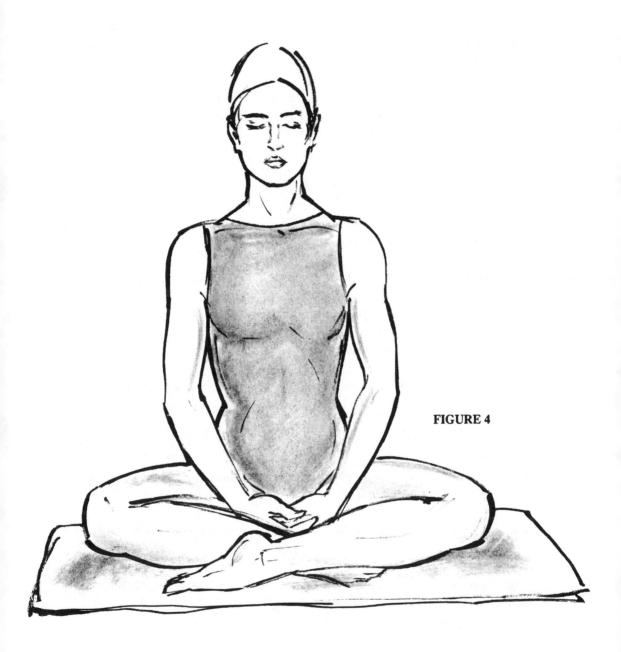

FIGURE 4

129

MORE SLEEP TIPS

Always sleep with your body aligned in an East/West Direction, with your head ideally facing towards the East. This insures that your energy is not drained by the earth's magnetic field.

Soft beds exert an enervating influence on you, and make the deep sleep we need more difficult to obtain. A thin padding, made out of a non-synthetic material, covered by a cotton sheet is good.

Use a pillow when sleeping at night. This keeps the blood circulating evenly. For short naps keep your feet slightly elevated.

Rising before the sun will help you conserve energy that otherwise would be drained by the earth's magnetic field.

The following exercises can increase and balance your energy upon getting up.

Cat Stretch: On your back. Bend your right knee to the outside of the left leg as you turn your upper body to the right. Stretch. Switch sides. This adjusts your magnetic field to separate you from sleep.

Stretch Pose: Head and heels six inches. Stare at your toes. Breath of Fire (this can be preceded by Bridge Pose). This adjusts your Navel Center.

Tuck Pose: Wrap your arms around your bent knees. Tuck your nose in between your knees. Breath of Fire. Then rock on your spine. Sit on your heels and lower your forehead to the ground. These exercises help your metabolism and eliminate gas.

Rub the soles of the feet and palms of the hands together. Create a heat. This stimulates your nerves.

Eagle Pose: Raise your arms to 60 degrees with the fingers curled into the palms facing forward, and thumbs pointing straight up. Breath of Fire. This strengthens your magnetic field.

Now, keep your feet bare and go to the bathroom sink. Turn the cold water on and off a few times. This grounds the electrical charge in the body.

Using a mixture of 2 parts potassium alum to 1 part salt (contact you local yoga Teacher for more information on this mixture), massage the back of your tongue with your toothbrush or finger (be careful) until you gag, and bring up mucous to be spit out. This mucous, which collects in the throat overnight, will eventually clog up your colon if not eliminated. This gagging reflex also causes your eyes to water, and is said to prevent cataracts.

Massage yourself with cold-pressed almond oil. This will give important nutrients to the skin and draw toxins out of the pores.

Take a cold shower, massaging yourself vigorously where the water hits. Use lukewarm for washing purposes and end with cold.

Drink a few glasses of water and do a yoga set and meditation.

Now you're ready to go about the day in a great way!

AND BEFORE BED:

Wash your feet in cold running water, brush your hair forward and back a few times (a wooden comb or natural bristles are best), and drink warm milk or bancha tea (both have a high calcium content .

CHAPTER 15 - GET DOWN TO GET UP

Depression has been called the "common cold of mental disorders." Close to 20% all Americans experience some form of chronic depression. Depression could be defined as a kind of debilitating malaise which makes life's stresses seem overwhelming and life's challenges insurmountable. Many people in the throes of depression use the phrase, "Unable to see the light at the end of the tunnel," to describe how they're feeling.

Depression manifests not only as sadness and grief, but can be characterized by insomnia, eating disorders, and a host of other physical symptoms i.e. constipation, headaches, dry skin, fatigue, fluctuating blood pressure, mood swings, and irritability.

Many forms of depression have been linked to a chemical imbalance in the brain. Currently there are a number of nutritional supplements which are being used to treat depression.

Proper diet as a tool towards lessening the severity of depression cannot be overemphasized. In recent years, hypoglycemia and Candida have been found to figure prominently as contributing factors in the diagnosis of depression.

From a yogic standpoint, the ultimate cause for depression is a lack of communication with one's creative essence. By this I mean soul, spirit, Divine aspect, that energy source which allows your inner life to become your outer expression. The techniques in this chapter can help you get your energy flowing again and remind you that you are a you! Your identity is Infinity and that's grounds for ecstasy!

The following sequence will get your energy flowing. Sometimes when you're feeling depressed, the best medicine is to simply move! This set is also specifically for athletes. It'll give you energy and endurance, and can be used as a prelude to any kind of athletic endeavor. In addition I have included two additional meditation techniques which can help you delete your depression

1. Sit on your heels with your knees wide. Interlace your fingers behind your neck, with your elbows pressed back. Breathe long and deeply through your nose for 3-5 minutes. Inhale and hold the breath for 5 seconds.

2. Frog Pose (figure 1). The heels are together and off the ground. Your arms are inside the knees, and you're supporting yourself with your fingertips. As you inhale straighten your knees and lower your head. As you exhale return to the original position (figure 2). Do 26 of these.

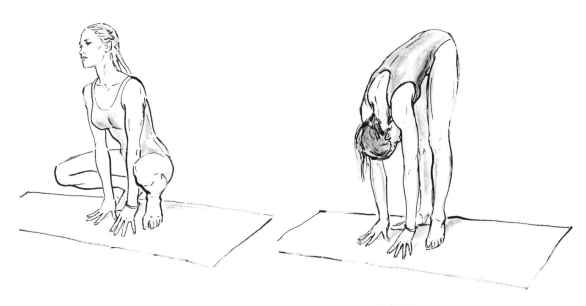

FIGURE 2   **FIGURE 1**

3. Immediately sit on your heels and do *Sat Kriya*. Your arms are extended up, so that the upper arms are hugging the ears. Your fingers are interlaced with the index fingers extended (figure 3). Say *Sat* as you pull your navel in. Say *Nam* as you relax your navel. Feel *Sat* deep inside your belly. Feel *Nam* rising up the spine. Do this for 11/2 minutes.

4. Do 10 frog pose.

5. Do *Sat Kriya* for 30 seconds.

6. Do Frog Pose 15 times.

7. Do *Sat Kriya* for 30 seconds.

8. Do Frog Pose slowly, with deep breaths, 10 times.

9. Come into position for *Sat Kriya*. Inhale, exhale, hold the breath out and apply Root Lock. Repeat. Relax.

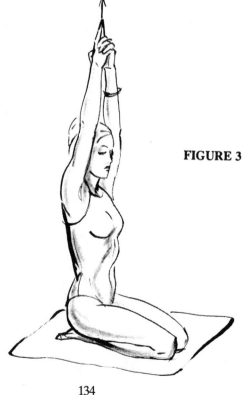

FIGURE 3

134

10. The following technique can be practiced as an exercise unto itself when you're feeling down. It's called *Maha Shakti Kriya*.

Extend your legs in front of you. Raise up into Cantilever Pose, your arms are parallel to the ground, and your legs are at a 60 degree angle in relation to the ground (figure 4). Inhale and hold the breath, as you press the back of your tongue against the roof of the mouth, and apply Root Lock. Hold the breath as long as you comfortably can. Exhale lower the legs. Repeat this exercise as many times as you'd like.

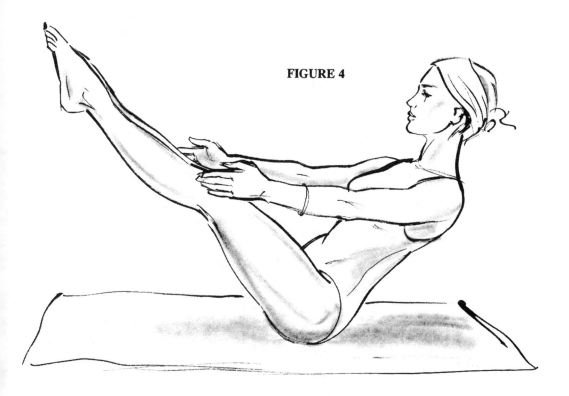

FIGURE 4

11. The following breath meditation can alleviate depression by balancing your brain hemispheres. The brain hemispheres frequently need to be rebalanced when a person has a history of drug use. In addition, it increases your lung capacity, which in turn can help you to feel more connected to the flow of life inherent in the breath.

Sitting with a straight spine. Your hands are in Gyan Mudra, the index fingers and thumbtips are meeting. With your upper arms parallel to the ground, bend your elbows so that the hands form "eyeglasses" over the eyes.

Throughout the first part of the meditation keep your eyes open. As you inhale press your elbows back somewhat as the hands separate and move out to the sides (figure 5). As you exhale return to the original position (figure 6). On the initial inhale think *Sa*. As you exhale think *Ta*. On the second inhale think *Na* on the second exhale think *Ma*. Do this slowly with a deep breathing for 2-3 minutes. Then increase the speed for 3 more minutes.

Now, with your hands in your lap, and the arms and shoulders relaxed, close your eyes and turn your eyes to the top of the head. Have no thoughts, simply bring your entire awareness to the highest elevation of the skull.

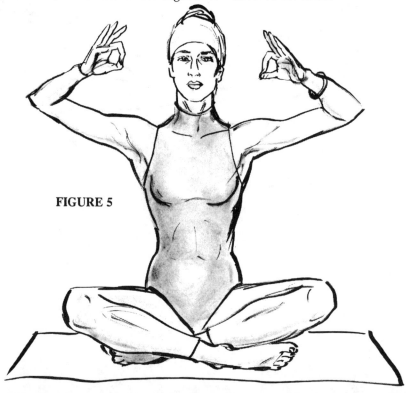

FIGURE 5

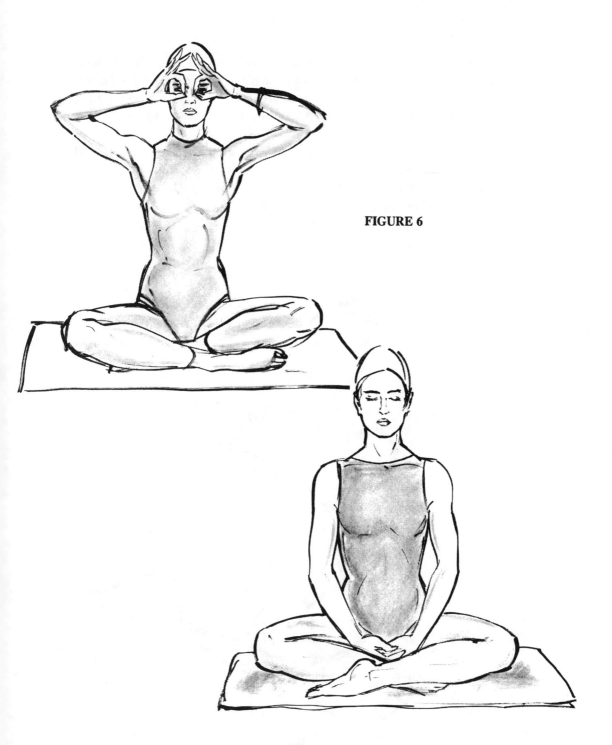

FIGURE 6

11. Sit comfortably with a straight spine. Your elbows are bent, the forearms are parallel to the ground. The backs of your hands are pressed together, at a level between the upper sternum and collarbone. The fingertips are pointing forward, and the thumbs are stretched, pointing straight down (figure 7).

Your eyes are 1/10th open looking down towards the tip of the nose. Inhale and chant the mantra *Wahay Guru* 16 times. Continue to chant *Wahay Guru* 16 times per breath, for 11 minutes. You can ultimately build this up to 31 minutes, and *Wahay Guru* 52 times per breath.

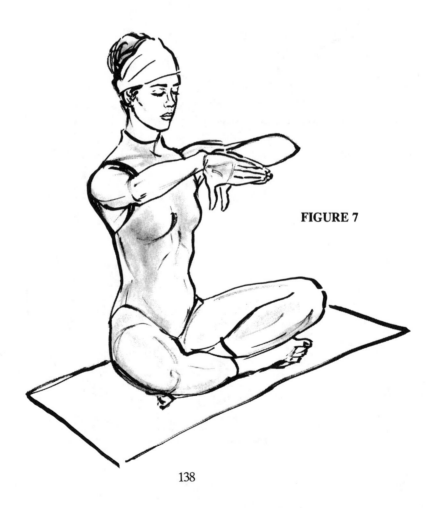

FIGURE 7

138

CHAPTER 16 - DIVING FOR THE BLUE PEARL

Creativity entails more than simply writing a poem, or painting a painting; it's also the applied intelligence, and intuitive capability which enables us to stay one step ahead of time and space. It's a personal statement stamped onto everything we do and are, the gifts we've been given to grow by, to heal and uplift others in powerful and original ways.

Creativity is linked to consciousness. In this work we raise our consciousness. That means we extend our ability to perceive subtle information from our inner and outer environments, and learn to trust and act in accordance with the Universe, or God if you will, the Ultimate Author, and Fashioner of all Forms.

In a physiological sense, creativity can be a reality when we've balanced, and are able to access the appropriate brain areas, the pituitary and pineal glands have been activated, and most importantly, when we've transcended our fears and inhibitions with the knowledge and awareness that our lives are open books wherein the particulars of a Destiny can be written.

We shall liberate our hungers
And transform them,
Crafting chaos in Freedom
And emotion in fiery Devotion,
And take a hammer to the house of mirrors,
And a writ of certainty to the casino of the world.

- Ravi Singh

The following techniques will serve as a terrific underpinning for any project, the successful outcome of which, depends on your inspiration and resourcefulness

1. Sit in a comfortable pose with your spine straight. Block your right nostril with the right thumb. The fingers of the right hand point straight up. Breathe long and deeply through the left nostril for 3 minutes (figure 1). As you inhale visualize and feel the light of the breath going down the left side of the spine. As you exhale feel it rise up the center of the spine.

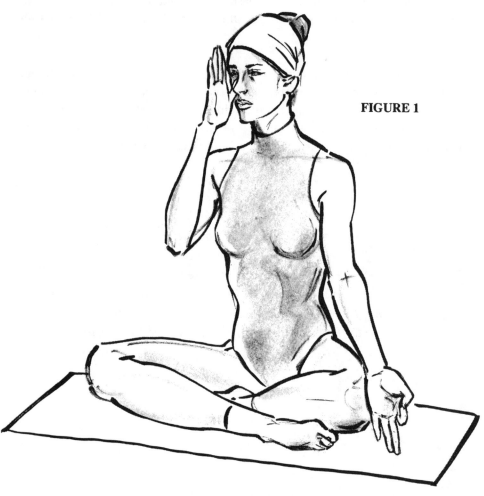

FIGURE 1

2 Sit on your heels and lower your forehead to the ground. Extend your arms straight out in front of you along the floor with the palms pressed together (figure 2). This pose in itself will bring circulation to the brain. That in turn, will engender clarity.

Inhale and hold the breath. Visualize the colors of the spectrum forming up the spine. Red at the base. Orange at hip level. Gold-yellow at the stomach and solar-plexus level. Spring green between the shoulder blades. Azure blue at throat level. Electric blue at the brow. Violet at the top of the head.

Now exhale and let the colors blend and explode into white. It's as if you're seeing yourself from a point above. Practice this for as long as you'd like.

FIGURE 2

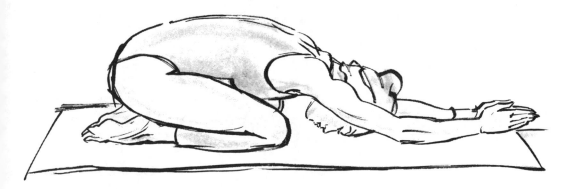

3. *Many creative blocks stem from an imbalance at the Throat Center. For instance, it's been postulated that the use of marijuana disrupts the flow of cerebral-spinal fluid (and thus energy) through the neck area, and base of the skull. Many marijuana abusers revel in the world of ideas, but lose the ability to carry them out.*

The following sequence works on the Throat Center, the seat of expression. The throat center relates to the element ether. It helps us create form out of formula, and being out of nothingness, so that we can give substance to idea.

A. Sit in a comfortable position with your spine straight. Your arms are at right angles with the upper arms parallel to the ground. The index fingers and thumbtips are meeting.

As you inhale turn your head left as straighten your elbows, so that the arms are parallel to the ground (figure 3). Exhale and turn your head right, bringing your arms back to the original position. (figure 4) 3 minutes.

B. Sit on your heels. Lean back 30 degrees. Drop your head back. Your eyes are open looking straight up, unblinking. Your arms are parallel to the ground, shoulder width apart, palms facing the ceiling. (figure 5) Breath of Fire 3 minutes.

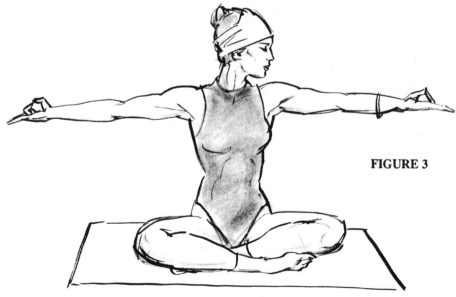

FIGURE 3

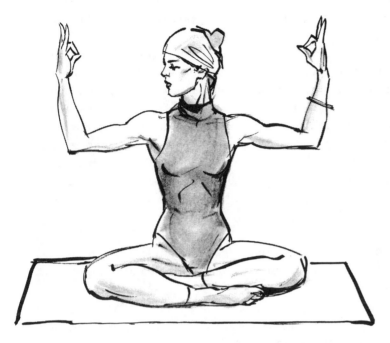

FIGURE 4

FIGURE 5

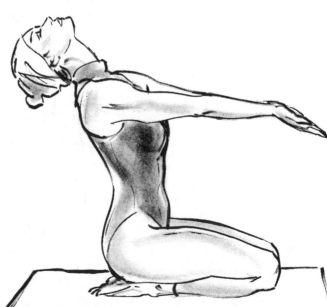

143

D. Still on your heels. Drop your head forward. Interlace your fingers at the small of the back, and pull your arms up. (figure 6) Breath of Fire 3 minutes.

E. The following breath meditation works on your Throat Center and metabolism to stimulate creativity. Sit in any comfortable position with your spine straight. Raise your arms to shoulder level, parallel to the ground. Bend your elbows, so that your hands are in front of your throat. Your hands are in fists, with the index and middle fingers extended. Your thumbs are folded over the down-turned ring and little fingers. The extended fingers are meeting tip to tip at throat level. Index to index, middle to middle. (figure 7) Inhale for 3 seconds, hold the breath for 5 seconds, and exhale slowly for 10-15 seconds. Continue this breathing pattern with sensitivity and control for up to 11 minutes.

F. Here's another breathing exercise guaranteed to stimulate creativity. It's *Sitali Pranayam*. Inhale through a curled tongue and exhale through your nose (figure 8). Time open.

It's said if you practice this exercise the heavens will serve you, meaning that by harnessing the element ether (associated with the Throat Center) whatever you conceive of will be granted. You'll be a master manifester.

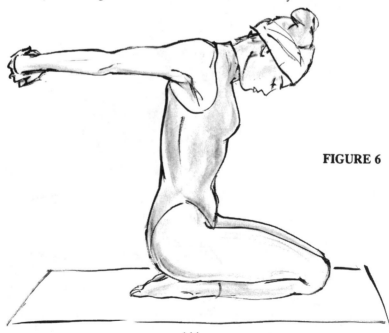

FIGURE 6

144

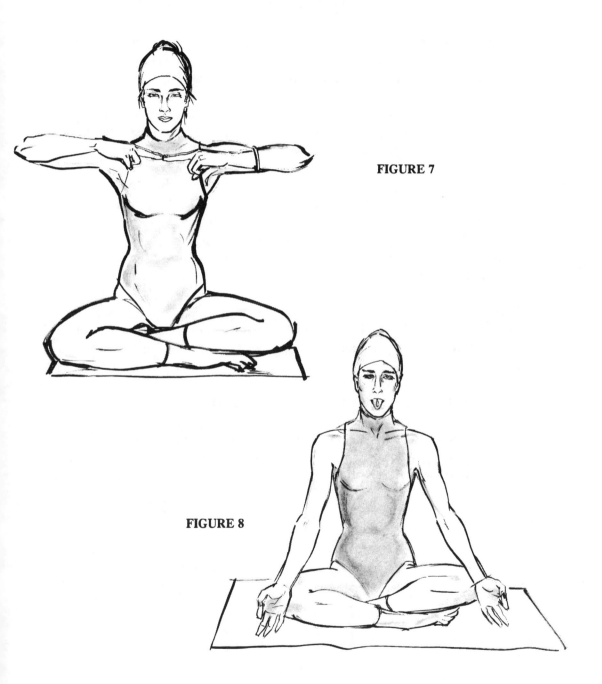

FIGURE 7

FIGURE 8

145

CHAPTER 17 - LONG LIVE YOU!

We as humans have the longest lifespan of any mammal on earth. Even so aging is frequently equated with loss of one's faculties, and clarity, being put out to pasture so to speak. This standard model lacks dignity at best.

Time is an insidious saboteur. It sneaks up on you by slow degrees. The time to halt the machinations of time is now. Through the appropriate lifestyle considerations and disciplines, you can live longer, look better, and forego a fate in favor of a Destiny.

Longevity depends on the health of the glands, the ability of the cells regenerate themselves (nutritional supplements classified as anti-oxidants seem to be a very important factor in this), the health of your immune system, and especially a love of life which keeps you open to new ideas and opportunities to expand and grow.

Recent research has shown that consciously restricting your caloric intake you move into your 30's and beyond can be an important factor in increasing longevity. Many yoga practitioners fast one day a week, to give their systems a rest and a boost.

Some people get injections from an extract of sheep embryos or go to expensive spas to try and turn back the clock on aging. Do it the yoga way! Without a doubt, if you make the techniques in this book a steady part of your life, there's no way you won't stay younger longer. Use these sets to prepare for your next high school reunion. You'll astound and amaze your peers!

The following exercises will strengthen your immunity system, detoxify you, help your body regenerate, and give you a powerful infusion of energy. The yogic claim for this set is, if you practice it honestly, it can "Heal anything that ails you."

In the following exercises, if you feel yourself starting to panic while holding the breath out, relax. Hold the breath out longer than you thought you could. You're working through your deepest fears, and helping your body to regenerate and heal at an accelerated rate.

1. Lie on your back. Raise your head and heels 6 in. off the ground. Have your hands under your buttocks palms facing down (figure 1). Inhale, exhale hold the breath out as long as you can while applying Root Lock. Inhale when you have to, exhale, and continue this breathing pattern. 3 minutes.

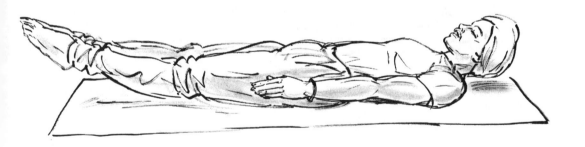

FIGURE 1

2. Lie on your stomach. Place your hands (in fists with the thumbs inside the fists) under the hips, in the cavity where the thighs meet the body. Your chin is on the ground, with your face facing forward. With the heels together, raise both legs off the ground (figure 2).

Exhale completely, apply Root Lock, and hold the breath out and as long as you can. Inhale when you must and exhale once more. Continue this cycle for up to 3 minutes.

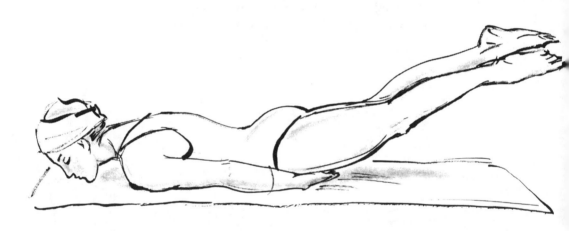

3. Lie on your back. Swing your legs up into Shoulder Stand. Support your lower back with your hands. Press your chin against the collarbone.

Exhale hold the breath out and kick your buttocks with alternate heels (figure 3). Continue this cycle, kicking your buttocks with the breath held out for up to 3 minutes. When you inhale, you can straighten your legs up before resuming the kicking. Be vigorous, it's not easy but it's glorious, so be victorious, in this endeavor to live forever!

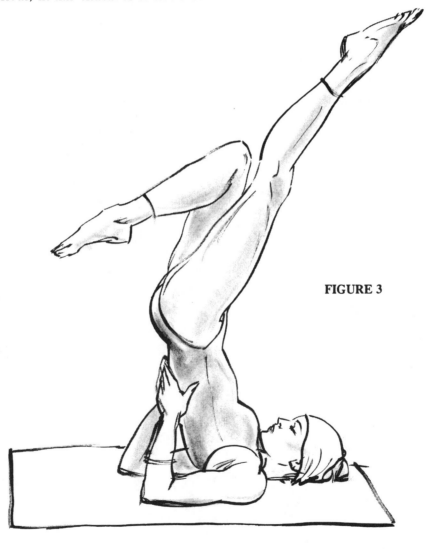

FIGURE 3

4. On your stomach again. Your hands are under the shoulders palms facing down, as if you're going to do a push-up. Come up into Cobra Pose (figure 4). Exhale, hold the breath out and apply *Mul Bhand*. Continue this cycle for up to 3 minutes. Relax.

FIGURE 4

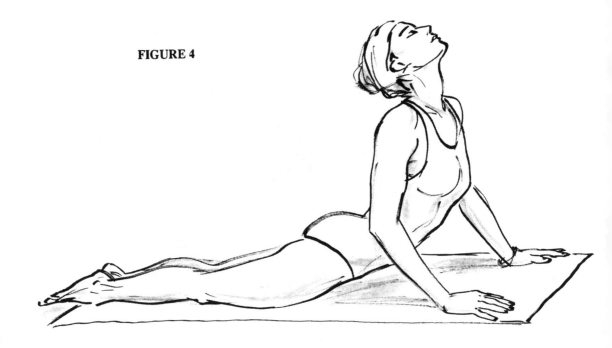

CHAPTER 18 - BEAUTY FROM WITHIN

Women are becoming increasingly aware that "beauty" is a total package in which nutrition, exercise, and concept of self, play major roles. In this process of self-discovery, many women are using the science of yoga to help them become healthy, happy, and fulfilled.

I think most people would agree that our culture has overstated the outer. The truly liberated woman recognizes that beauty is a power of positive projection, an appreciation of her own mystery, dignity, divinity, grace, and strength. Essentially a woman's inner environments make her what she is.

Being the owner of a feminine vehicle entails a responsibility, which requires bringing balance to the many facets of you. The crux of this is a healthy glandular and nervous system, good circulation of energy and blood, and the cultivation of confidence, creativity, and charisma.

I asked the actress Linda Thorson, who's been practicing Kundalini Yoga for 6 years, to discuss the concept of beauty in light of her own experience. "In my life, beauty is based on lack of fear, the ability to relax, and in allowing myself to be successful with no compulsion or compromise. I became secure with my beauty when I realized it was unique, and at the same time part of what women are in essence."

You as a woman should take time every day to meditate and relax. In your totality you're a rare instrument upon which the most sublime and beautiful music can be played. It must cared for though, and kept in tune.

Yoga philosophy sees the essence of Woman as *Adi Shakti*, the Feminine Creative Principle, Divine Mother, Primal Power, energy of the Universe. Kundalini, the energy of spirit rising, is considered to be a manifestation of this.

It's said that a woman's heartfelt prayer can move heaven and earth, and that her compassion can bring hope to the hopeless and ease all sorrow.

What follows is a breath meditation for metabolic balancing, exercises for daily maintenance, an exercise for beauty, and dietary and lifestyle considerations, specifically for women.

Also included is a meditation for women only, which can serve as an effective tool to help you keep your emotions in perspective, maintain a relationship with your creative self, and become radiant and resourceful.

One Smile from you
Is worth a thousand words.
One look from you
Can change destinies
Into blessings from God.
One touch from you
Can heal and sustain.
O woman if you just be kind
There will be no more tears
On this earth.

-Yogi Bhajan

1. The following breath meditation can calm the nerves and bring about hormonal balance. If practiced regularly it can help a woman adjust her menstrual cycle. Sit up straight with the wrists on the knees, palms facing slightly up (figure 1).

Inhale in 4 equal parts, and exhale in one. As you inhale in 4 parts, press your thumbtips against successive fingertips - index, middle, ring, and little. As you exhale in one part bring your thumb back to the index finger.

As you inhale think the sounds *Sa Ta Na Ma*, as you exhale think *Wahay Guru*. Your eyes are 1/10 open, gazing down towards the tip of the nose. Press the back of your tongue against the roof of your mouth. The teeth are pressed together. Try this for 3-11 minutes. Ultimately you can work up to 31 minutes. To end inhale, hold the breath, keeping your tongue pressed up.

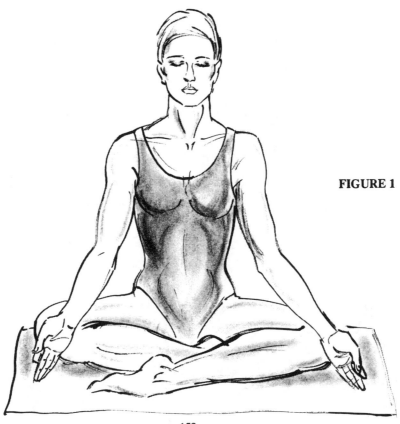

FIGURE 1

YOGA POSES FOR DAILY MAINTENANCE

These yoga poses can be done as a "set" or individually throughout the day.

2. Archer Pose (figure 2). Standing, have your feet a little more than shoulder width apart. Turn the left foot so that the toes are pointing to the left. Shift the right heel 3 inches to the right. Bend your left knee keeping your right leg straight. Your left arm is extended straight, while your right arm is bent at the elbow, the right hand is next to the right ear. Both hands are in fists.

Stare out over the extended arm. Breath long and deeply. You're working on the nerves to be calm in a crisis. Do this for 1-3 minutes then switch sides.

3. Life Nerve Stretch (figure 3). With both legs extended straight, hold your toes, ankles, calves, or knees. Long Deep Breathing 1-3 minutes.

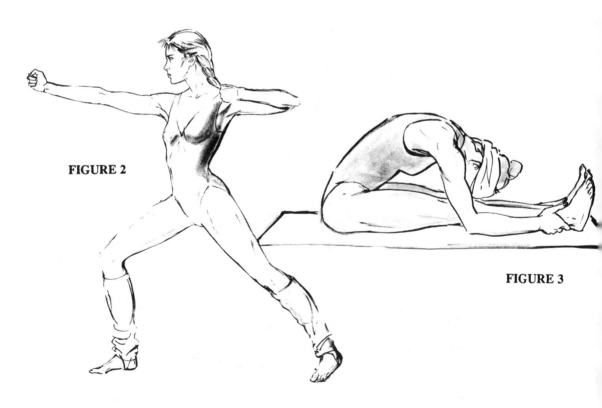

FIGURE 2

FIGURE 3

4. Camel Pose: From a kneeling position, reach back and grab your ankles or heels. Press your hips forward and let your head drop back. If your lower back feels put upon modify the exercise (figure 4). Hold this pose for 1-3 minutes with Long Deep Breathing.

Camel Pose can be instrumental in preventing buildup of tension around the ovaries (this in turn may be a factor in lessening the severity of problems such as menstrual cramps and ovarian cysts. It also works on the lymphatic system and constitutes an anti-breast cancer measure.

5. Baby Pose. Sit on your heels and lower your forehead to the ground. The arms are along the sides with the palms facing up by the ankles. Feel very secure, very pure, and relax in this pose for as long as you'd like.

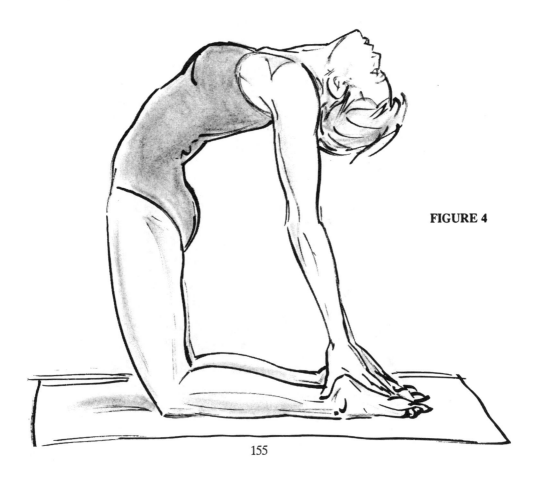

FIGURE 4

6. Stretch Pose (figure 5). Lay on your back with your heels 6 inches off the ground. Stare at your toes. Breath of Fire 1-3 minutes.

7. Bow Pose (figure 6) Lie on your stomach. Reach back and hold your ankles. Flex your feet. Raise your thighs and upper body off the floor. Breath of Fire 1-3 minutes.

Bow Pose with Breath of Fire will trim the waistline, system, and adjust the navel pulse.

FIGURE 5

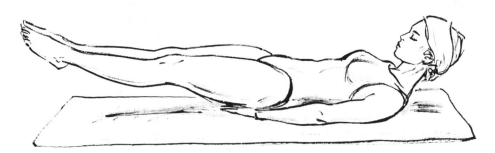

FIGURE 6

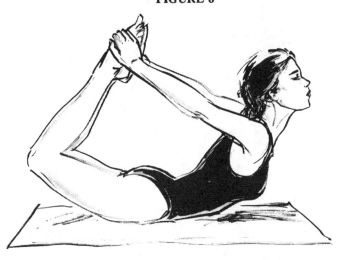

8. Shoulder Stand (figure 7) Swing your legs up and support your lower back with your hands. Press your chin firmly against the collar bone, and use your elbows and arms to give you a firm foundation. Hold with Long Deep Breathing for as long as you'd like.

Shoulder Stand realigns the internal organs (which literally get displaced by the pull of gravity), increases circulation to the brain for clarity and deep rest, tonifies the kidneys, assists in the prevention of varicose veins, and stimulates the thyroid gland for metabolic balance.

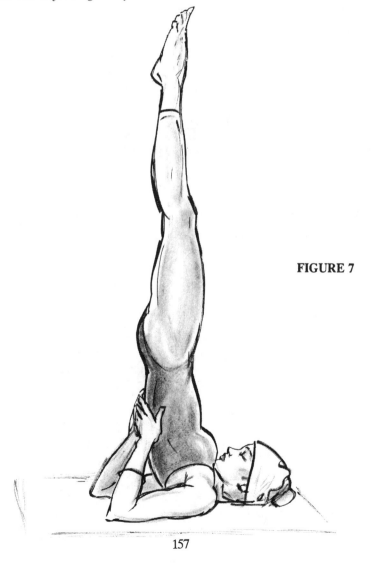

FIGURE 7

157

9. Cow Pose (figure 8). On your hands and knees. Press your head up, and your stomach towards the ground. Focus at the brow. Breath of Fire 3-5 minutes.

Cat Pose (figure 9) Drop your head and curve your spine. Continue Breath of Fire for 3-5 minutes more.

These two poses, in conjunction with the Breath of Fire, can help you balance your glandular system. The glands are the guardians of your beauty, and mental and physical health and well-being.

FIGURE 8

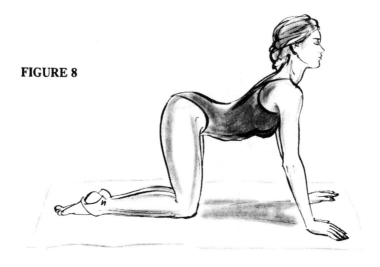

FIGURE 9

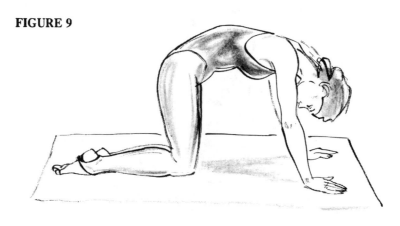

10. *Sat Kriya* (figure 10) Sit on your heels. Raise your arms up so that the upper arms are hugging the ears. As you say *Sat* pull your navel in towards the spine. As you say *Nam* relax the navel and feel the sound move up the spine. Continue for 3 minutes. To end inhale hold the breath and apply Root Lock. Then hold the breath out and squeeze up. Inhale and relax.

11. Relax on your back and let yourself go.

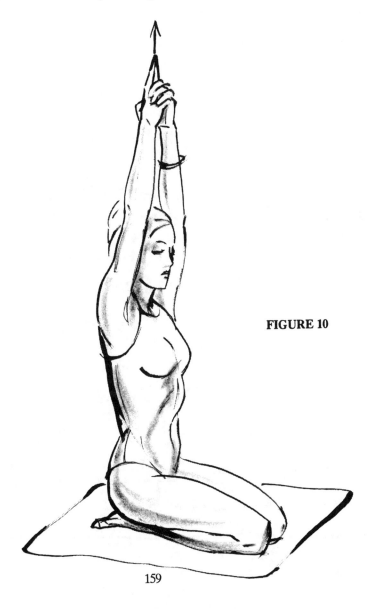

FIGURE 10

12. Sit on your heels. Interlace your fingers at the small of the back. Pull your hands off your back, and angle forward. Keep your head up and face facing forward (figure 11). Inhale and hold the breath as long as you comfortably can. As you hold the breath stretch the arms up. Do this up to 4 times.

This exercise is for beauty. It brings a lot of circulation into the face and helps your immune system.

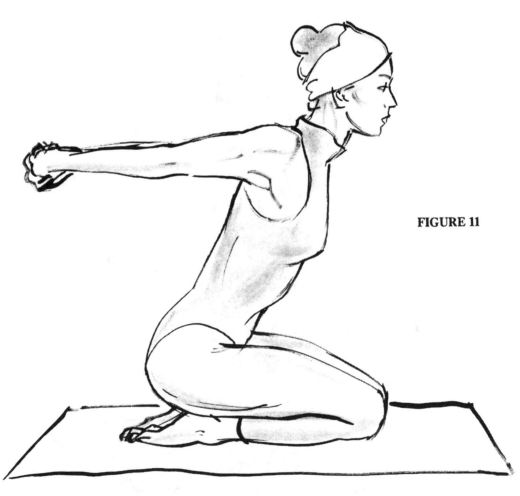

FIGURE 11

13 Sit up straight. Block your right nostril with your right thumb. The other fingers are pointing straight up (figure 12). Inhale deep through the left nostril and hold the breath as long as you comfortably can. Exhale through the right nostril, and hold the breath out as long as you comfortably can. Time open.

This breath meditation is an effective self-help therapy which can help you overcome compulsive habit patterns, and ease stress. This technique can be very effective if you're trying to stick to a diet, quit smoking, or lessen anxiety.

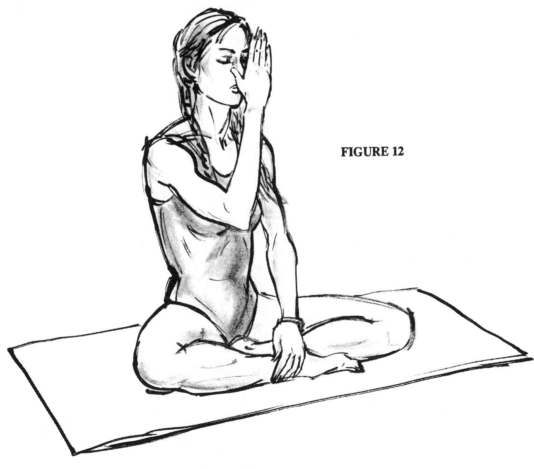

FIGURE 12

14. Lie on your stomach, with the arms along the sides, palms facing up. Your face is facing forward, chin on the floor (figure 13). Press your thumbtips against successive fingertips.

As you press your thumbs against the index fingertips think *Sa*. As you press your thumbs against the middle fingertips think *Ta*. As you press your thumbs against the ring fingertips think *Na*. As you press your thumbs against the little fingertips think *Ma*.

Do this for 11-31 minutes anytime. You can even do it before getting out of bed in the morning or before sleep.

This meditation can help you balance your emotions and make you graceful and great.

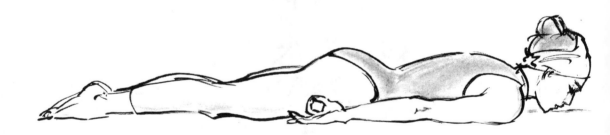

FIGURE 13

LIFESTYLE CONSIDERATIONS FOR WOMEN

To maintain your health and beauty you should eat food that clears your stomach in 2 hours and is digested and eliminated within 18 hours.

For beauty's sake avoid heavy meals, alcohol, smoking, caffeine, and meat.

For inner cleansing and proper ph, try douching with a mixture of 1 part homemade or plain yogurt to ten parts water. You can also add a little tumeric (the spice that makes mustard yellow). Do this for 4 days before your period, and three days after.

If you feel fatigued during your period take a teaspoon of cold-pressed sesame seed oil daily during your cycle, and for a few days afterwards.

If you're menstruating more than normal and/or if the flow is too thick, take lecithin, vitamin E, and milk in which black peppercorns have been boiled.

To lessen the intensity of menstrual cramps, steep 4 or 5 slices of fresh ginger and drink as tea.

To replace minerals lost during your cycle, saute 1~16 almonds in almond oil or ghee (clarified butter). Make this part of your breakfast each day of your cycle.

Many women in our culture begin to show symptoms of menopause as early as age 36. Chances are if you exercise regularly, and keep your diet sensible, you can forego this transition until much later in life, and lessen its severity.

To compensate for the loss of estrogen after menopause begins take vitamin E, liquid chloryphyll (women of all ages should take this daily), and up to an ounce of cold-pressed almond oil each day. Use almond oil in salad dressings or in the recipe which follows. (According to yoga, almond oil can help lower your cholesterol level, break down fat, keep your skin aglow, and assist in stabilizing blood sugar levels).

A great breakfast drink for women: Take 1 ripe banana, 8 ounces of orange juice, 1 tablespoon of liquid chloryphyll, 2 teaspoons of rice bran syrup, and 2 teaspoons of cold-pressed almond or sesame seed oil. Blend until frothy You may find that this in itself will tide you over until noon, when it's most prudent to have your most substantial meal of the day.

Get into the habit of exercising each day so that your sweat. Try and do yoga and exercise before you eat anything, first thing in the morning, as well as any other time which suits you.

And first thing before the first thing, take a cold shower. Now, I know this sounds extreme, but this practice can help you to become unbelievably healthy, and strong.

The procedure is this: massage yourself with almond oil and/or brush your skin with a loofa sponge. Then simply turn the cold water on and step into the shower, massaging yourself where the water hits. After about 5-10 seconds step out. Do this three more times. By the 4th time you won't even feel the cold.

Cold showers will build your resistance to colds, flu, and hayfever, give you strong nerves, and an overall glow, flush the capillaries, oxygenate the inner organs, help the tissues release pent-up toxins, and make you feel great! Afterwards, rub yourself briskly with a soft towel. You'll be suprised to find that you'll be a lot less sensitive to cold.

When you're having your period use lukewarm water. According to yogic lore, hot showers and baths will ultimately make your skin saggy and dull. For washing purposes lukewarm water is best.

CHAPTER 19 - MANPOWER

As men we are ruled by the sun (symbolic of a quality of energy) and should seek to emulate its qualities. It gives light equally to all (compassion), it illuminates (intelligence), and it never misses a day (firm in its commitments).

The real mark of a man is his constancy, the ability to establish and stick to his values and word, in the face of all odds and temptations. The true spirit of a man is his "Undying Infinite Potential."

As men, the key to our success lies in our ability to utilize our creative intelligence. All creativity is in fact sexual energy raised to a higher frequency. Kundalini Yoga can help us to "harness our horniness," and access our higher potential.

An important facet of our true strength is called the arcline, which is an aspect of our aura. The arcline helps us to project, protect, compute outside influences, and refute negativity. A strong arcline engenders a radar-like capacity which helps us to be somewhat invincible.

It's also an extension of the beaming power of our minds, and our prayerfulness, which translate into flow of spirit. With this flow of spirit as a constant, we can afford to be magnanimous, and thus we will be sought after and successful in all realms. Consistent meditation will give you this.

A man's spiritual path must be direct and uncompromising, although to complete it only two pre-requisites must be met: a man must live righteously and be Divine, in his communication, projection, commitments, creativity, and career. Everything he does must be in the Name of Truth, *Sat Nam!*

MENS' EXERCISES FOR POTENCY & POTENTIAL

1. First thing in the morning: lying on your back, bend your knees into your body so that your feet come off the ground. Move your knees to and from your head (figure 1) Do this 10-15 times.

This exercise will correct your lower back, and is very helpful for the elimination system.

2. Exercise #2 is also for your elimination system. It's also outlined in Chapter 7. Assume Baby Pose (figure 2). You're sitting on your heels with your forehead on the ground. The arms are along the sides, palms up. Move your buttocks side to side, as if your were a dinosaur thrashing its tail through the primordial wooods.

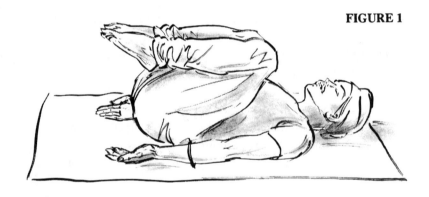

FIGURE 1

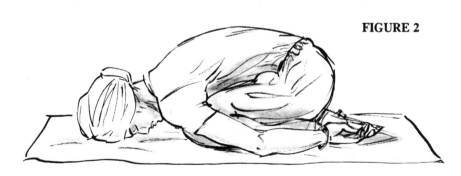

FIGURE 2

3. This next one also works on adjusting the hips. You need a prop, a bathroom sink will do. Grasp it firmly and put all your weight into it Arch your lower spine. Now step with the right foot across the left leg, and the reverse. Keep going for ten minutes. This will build your lower back (figure 3).

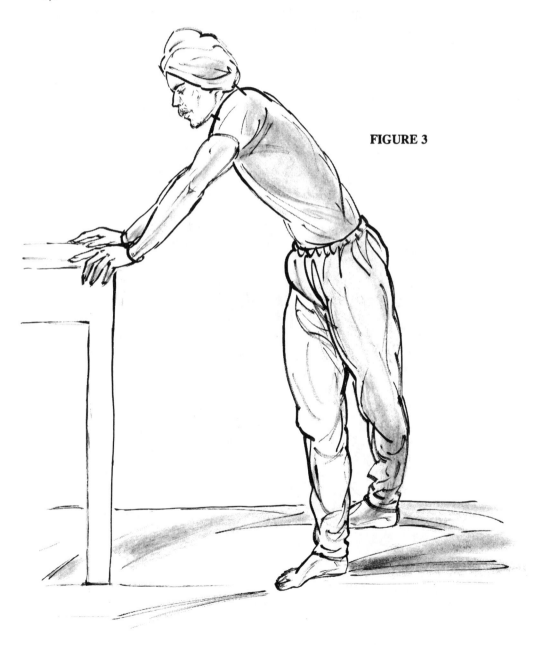

FIGURE 3

4. Chair Pose. For nerve strength and potency. Your feet are 2-3 ft. apart. Bend your knees, grab behind the ankles, and have your back parallel to the ground (figure 4). Breath of Fire 3 minutes.

Variation: With your back to the wall bend your knees so that your thighs are parallel, and calves perpendicular to the ground, press your lower back into the wall. Breath of Fire 3 minutes.

FIGURE 4

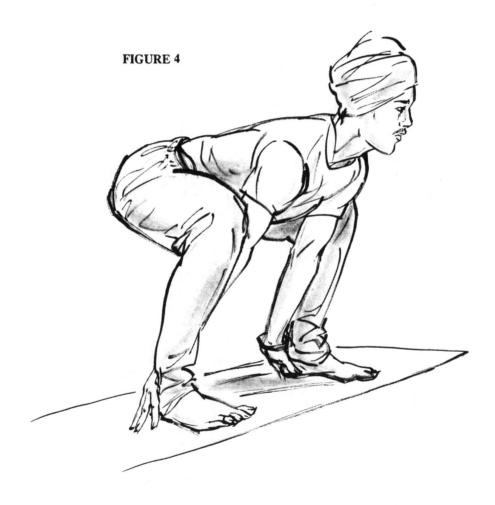

5. The yogic claim for the following exercise is that it revitalizes the sexual system and organs. Assume Crow Pose, squatting with your feet flat and knees bent (figure 5). In this variation hold the outside of your ankles. Breath of Fire 3 minutes.

6. This one's somewhat advanced, so be prudent. With the soles of the feet together, balance on the sides of the feet, with the knees off the ground. You're supporting yourself with your hands (figure 6). Bounce up and down with the Breath of Fire for 1 minute. Carefully come out of it.

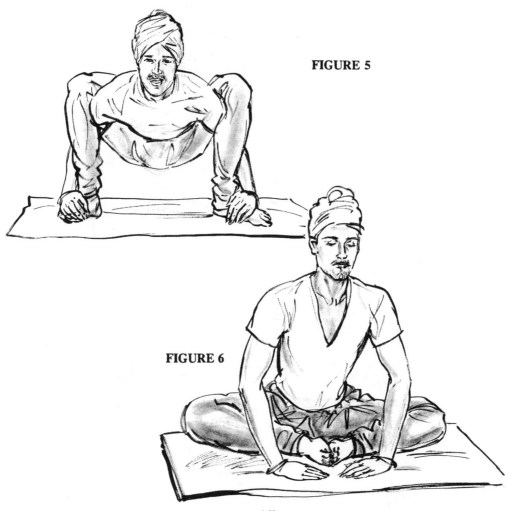

FIGURE 5

FIGURE 6

7. This exercise can be useful as a self-help therapy in treating certain sexual dysfunctions including premature ejaculation. Extend your legs straight and pull back on the toes. Elongate your spine, and pull your chin back like a soldier at attention (figure 7).

Inhale, exhale and hold the breath out. As you keep the breath expelled apply Root Lock. Inhale when you must and exhale immediately. Continue this cycle 8-26 times.

FIGURE 7

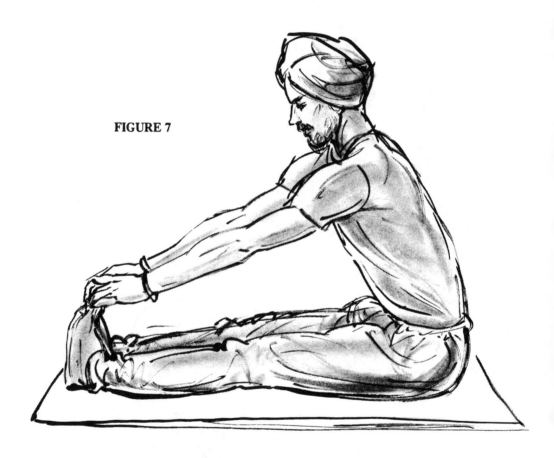

8. This one also works on potency and alleviates sexual dysfunctions. Come onto your hands and knees. Your head is up. Raise your right hand as if taking an oath (let it be, "I will do my best come what may."). Raise your left leg off the ground (figure 8).

Inhale and hold the breath, pump your left leg up and down 10 times, exhale, inhale and repeat. Do this 8 times, pumping the leg with the breath held. Move the leg as one unit from the hip socket. The leg stays off the ground throughout. Switch sides and repeat. Relax upon completion.

FIGURE 8

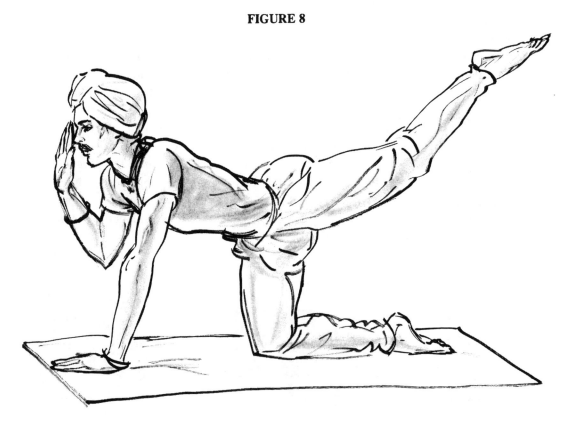

9. Stretch Pose. Lie on your back, raise your head and heels 6 inches (figure 9). Do Long Deep Breathing. In this variation you must hold the pose "until you shake." Stretch pose adjusts your navel center which has been described as the "creative nucleus of your potency." Relax after this one.

10. And now according to Yogi Bhajan, and his ancient illustrious predecessors, through whose sacrifice the integrity of the science of Kundalini Yoga has been maintained, this is the "Ultimate Man's Exercise." It's *Sat Kriya* in Full Lotus Pose (figure 10). Have each foot on the opposite thigh. Please don't force it!

(To increase your ability to sit in full lotus you can do the following: Extend your left leg straight. Put your right foot on the left thigh. Bounce your right knee up and down 26 times. Switch sides.)

Sitting in full lotus, or an approximate pose. Extend your arms up so that the upper arms hug the ears. Interlace your fingers with the index fingers extended. As you say *Sat* pull your navel in, as you say *Nam* relax your navel. Pulsate the sound between the navel and the brow. This is as much a mental exercise as a physical one. Continue for 3-31 minutes and relax equal to the time of the exercise.

VARIATION: Extend your right leg back, with the top of the foot on the ground. Your left foot is flat, with the left knee bent, and the left thigh parallel to the ground. Press your palms together with the fingers pointing straight (figure 11). Do *Sat Kriya* in this pose. As you say *Sat* pull your navel in, and as you say *Nam* relax your navel. If you have trouble keeping your balance, your eyes can be open staring straight.

FIGURE 9

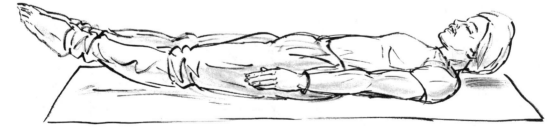

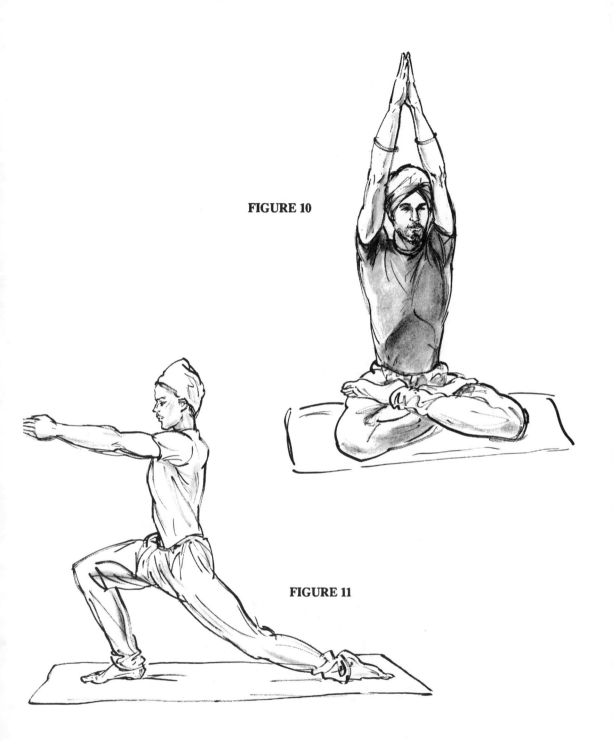

FIGURE 10

FIGURE 11

173

11. MEDITATION TO MAKE YOU GREAT

Sometimes as men we don't know our own strength, because the conditioning that helped forge our identity as men did not offer a strong and compassionate male model to emulate. Many of us were never told we have the capacity to excel. This breath meditation will help you increase your self-esteem and become confident, fearless, and great!

Sit in a comfortable pose with a straight spine. Interlace your fingers, and place your hands palms down over the solar plexus, at the base of the ribs (figure 12). Inhale, exhale, hold the breath out and mentally repeat the following 3 times:

Sat Narien, Wahay Guru, Hari, Narien Sat Nam

This means Clear Perception of Truth, Ecstasy Beyond Words, Clear Perception of the Creative Essence of the Divine, and Truth is God's Name. Say the sound slowly to yourself, so that you can extend the time you hold the breath out and work through your fears. 11 minutes.

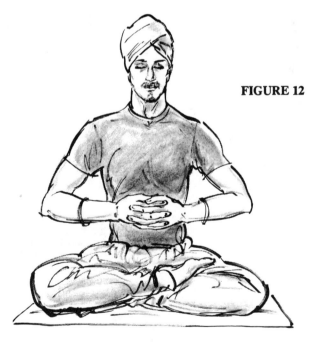

FIGURE 12

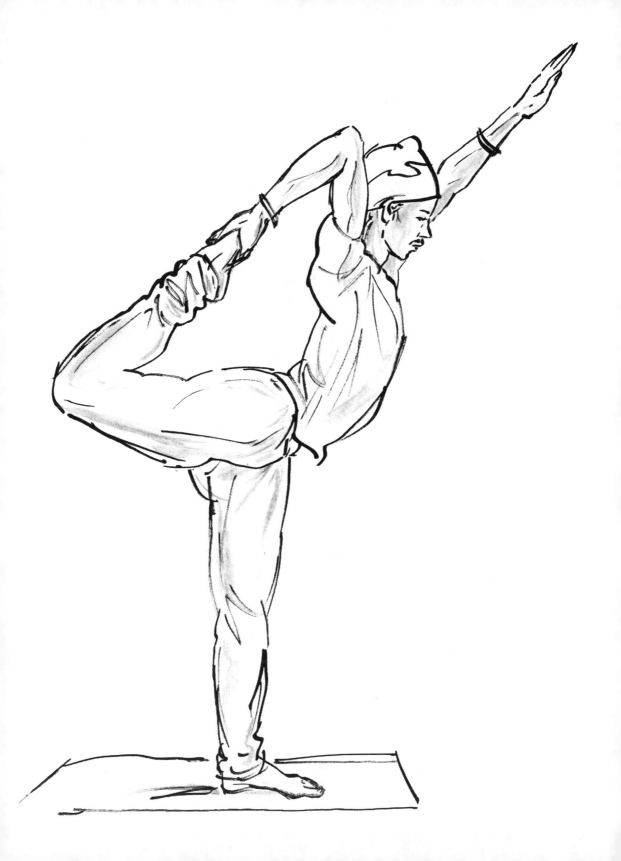

LIFESTYLE CONSIDERATIONS FOR MEN

The following lifestyle and dietary considerations will keep your male machine in gear:

Soft beds are an indulgence your back ultimately can't afford. It's best to sleep on a futon or mat.

A man should always urinate sitting down. According to yoga, this can prevent impotency in later years. Also, while urinating, you should stop the flow a few times, by contracting the urethra muscles. This will keep your sexual muscles in shape, and prevent the formation of kidney stones.

Ghee or clarified butter is a tonic for your nervous system and whenever possible, should be used in place of oil or butter. You can prepare *ghee* by boiling butter on a low flame and skimming off the white residue which coagulates on the surface. *Ghee* does not go rancid as butter does.

There are three "roots" which can keep you healthy on all levels. They are onion, garlic, and ginger. You can use them in any combination or context. They are called the trinity roots, the trident of life.

When your relationships, career, health, or mental outlook,are not up to par, you should do the following immediately: 1. Restrict your caloric intake, in other words, eat less. 2. Totally forswear all "heavy food," such as cheese, fried foods, meat, and sugar. 3. Cut out coffee, alcohol, and soda.

CHAPTER 20 - BEYOND SEX TOGETHER

Sex and relationship in the context of a conscious lifestyle should be approached with reverence and mutual respect. Your basic motive should always be, to relate to, and uplift the soul of your partner.

Marriage has been called the highest (and most difficult) yoga. Its success depends upon the ability of you and your partner to honor the Word, not a temporary fascination with a personality, but a promise given and accepted unto Infinity.

> *Marriage is a Heavenly Alliance,*
> *A Harmony of Hearts,*
> *Greater than the sum of its parts,*
> *A miracle of completion,*
> *A circle open to the sky,*
> *A prayerful partnership*
> *Stamped with Destiny's seal of approval,*
> *In which opposites salute the other*
> *In Eternity's deep embrace,*
> *And together as One*
> *Blend with the Light of the Long Time Sun.*

> --Ravi Singh

The following couples' exercises or Venus *Kriyas* are techniques whereby a man and woman can find a point of balance in relationship and learn to appreciate, support, and nurture one another's higher self. Remember, yoga is a microcosm of life. The sensitivity and strength you bring to these exercises will carry over into your life and allow your relationship to become a platform of elevation, a cup of blessings, and a path to Infinity.

Always remember to tune in together with *Ong Namo Guru Dev Namo* (see introduction). In addition, follow this by chanting:

Ad (odd) Guray Namay, Jugad Guray Namay,
Sat Guray Namay, Siri Guru Dev A Namay

This means: I bow to the Primal Wisdom, I bow to the Wisdom through the ages, I bow to the True Wisdom, I bow to the Great Invisible Wisdom

It's chanted in a monotone. This is a mantra of protection and reverence. Always remember to use the following exercises for righteous purposes only. They are powerful and should be respected.

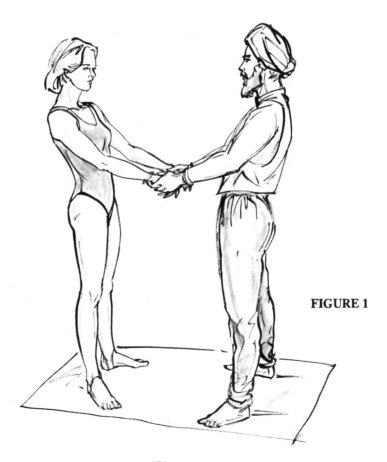

FIGURE 1

1. Sit on your heels facing your partner. Gaze into each other's eyes. Radiate love. See yourself in your partner's eyes. Continue for about 1 minute.

2. Stand up and join hands (figure 1). Inhale and exhale as you squat down. Hold the breath out for a few seconds. Inhale as you stand up and hold the breath for a few seconds (figure 2). Throughout the exercise gaze into each other's eyes. Do this one for about 1 minute.

FIGURE 2

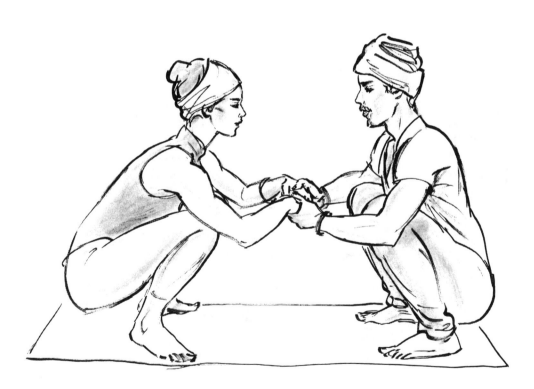

179

3. Extend your legs in front of you, with your feet sole to sole with your partner's. Keep your knees straight. Extend your arms and grasp your partner's hands. Inhale as one of the partners leans back, and exhale reverse (figure 3). Continue for about a minute, then relax.

FIGURE 3

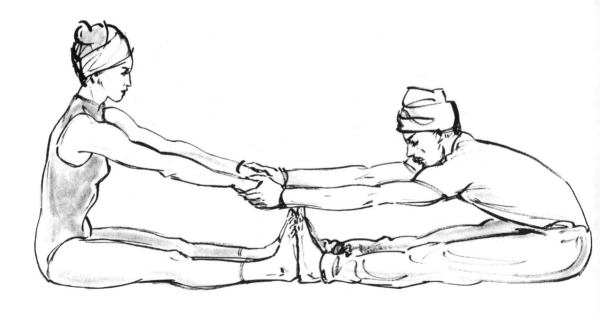

4. Again, with your feet meeting sole to sole with your partner's (and your essences meeting soul to soul!), extend your legs up and out, with your arms inside the legs, and the hands clasped (figure 4). You're balancing on your sacrums. Look eye to eye and do the Breath of Fire for up to 3 minutes. Inhale and apply Root Lock, Exhale and apply Root Lock again. Inhale and relax.

FIGURE 14

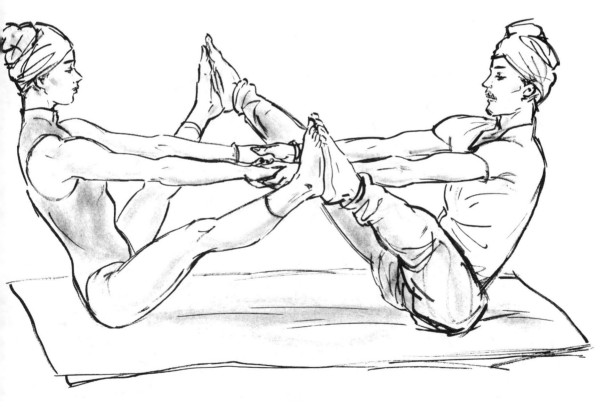

5. Sit in easy pose, across from your partner, knee to knee, and eye to eye. Your hands form a lotus. Your hands are cupped and the fingers are spread, with the little fingers and thumbs meeting along their lengths. The man puts his little fingers inside the woman's. This is the only point of contact. It's called Heart Lotus. (figure 5) Look into the soul and heart of your partner beaming love through your eyes. Continue for 11/2 minutes.

Now place your hands, one over the other on the sternum. (figure 6) Close your eyes and see your partner's eyes in your mind's eye. Go deep into your heart and find the source of unqualified love there. To end take a few deep breaths and relax.

6. Sit back to back with your partner and draw your knees up to your chest (figure 7). Meditate on your heart. Hear it. Meditate on the sun. Bring it into your heart and burn out any bitterness you've felt over the years. Continue for as long as you'd like.

FIGURE 5

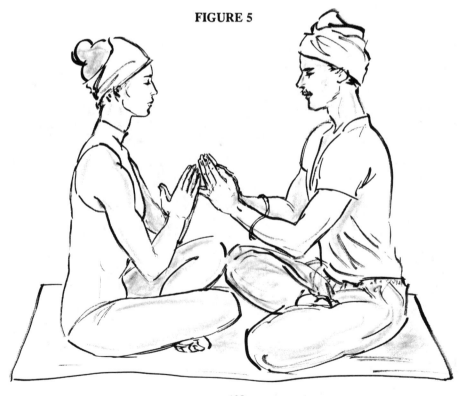

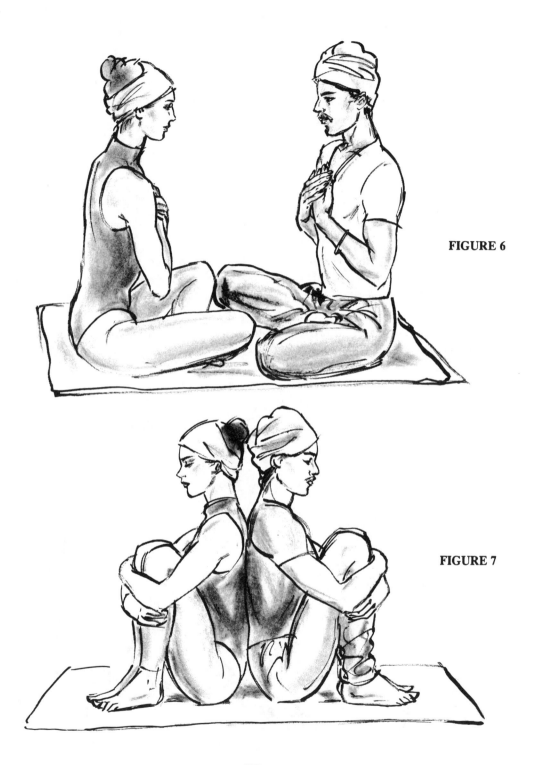

FIGURE 6

FIGURE 7

183

7. Sit facing each other knee to knee. Rest one hand in the other, both palms facing up, against the body at the base of the sternum. (figure 8) Focus at the brow. To begin the man inhales and chants:

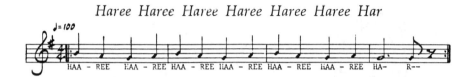

Haree Haree Haree Haree Haree Haree Har

As the man is chanting *Har* the woman inhales and then chants in response to the man. Chant very beautifully, to the heart of your partner, and listen to your polarity. As you do this focus at the brow and visualize the color green.

This meditation is for marital stability, communication from the heart, healing yourself and others, and prosperity. You can do this from 3-31 minutes.

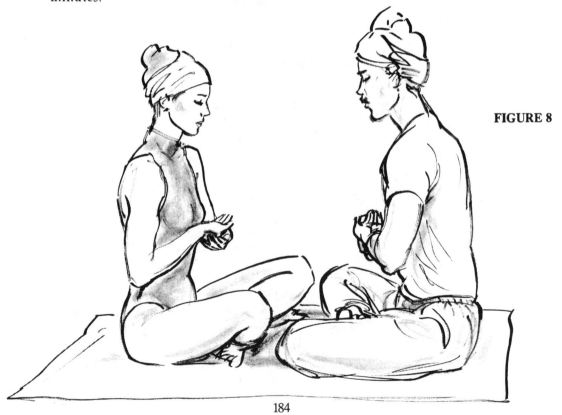

FIGURE 8

184

8. Another powerful couples exercise, is *Kirtan Kriya* (as outlined in chapter 21), practiced sitting back to back (figure 9).

FIGURE 9

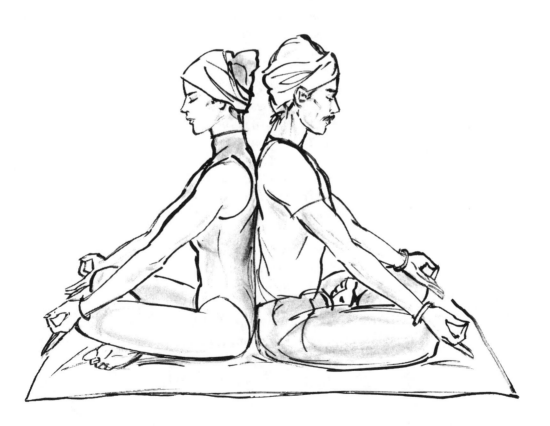

DATE WITH THE BELOVED

When I answered
The doorbell of the Infinite--
A paramour I longed for
Had come to call
With a bouquet of blessings,
And a searing love
Rent my heart
With lightning.

O Hero of All,
In your white convertible
Of Consciousness,
You showed me earth--
Planet on its axis of amnesia,
And all wonders
And all worlds,
As we hurtled through
This boundless and
Breathtaking firmament,
The beauty of your Creation
Became known to me,
And you consoled my soul
With a priceless gift,
The diamond pin of a Destiny!

One kiss from you
Fills the cave of my body
With light,
Fears clear
In the heaven of your embrace.
The pain of separation
Fades and is forgotten,
By your Power and by your Grace.

--Ravi Singh

CHAPTER 21 - THE INSIDE STORY

Infinity is not a place, it's an experience. Throughout history many people have found, to varying degrees, that the means to this experience is the process of meditation. In an immediate sense, this process can help us to become more alert and alive, it can also help us to develop our mental and intuitive faculties more effectively. Over time, meditation can help us gain the power of discernment, to help us make the most appropriate and responsible decisions, in matters concerning both our inner and outer lives

By practicing meditation, we want to eventually learn to unite with the object of our focus. In Kundalini Yoga and Meditation our focus is always an aspect of the Divine, towards the development of Divine attributes in ourselves .

Many people have the idea that meditation involves altered mental states, visions, trance states, and astral travels. While phenomena of this nature makes for interesting reading, it has very little to do initially, with the practical matters at hand.

The true process of meditation begins when we begin to confront and clear mental "garbage." What I mean by this is the accumulated stress of a lifetime, memories, fears, emotional scars, neuroses, and all the other subconscious debris which keeps us alienated from our essence.

Through dealing with our negativity, in the controlled environment of a meditation, we're to letting it get the best of us in our day to day lives.

Another erroneous assumption, on the part of many, is that there's only one type of meditation. The fact is, that there are thousands of different techniques, each of which work on a specific aspect of you.

By practicing the kinds of meditative techniques presented here, on a regular basis, you'll find that the patterns of your past will no longer subvert you. Everything in your life will become a spiritual exercise and take on a powerful significance.

Try practicing one or more of the following techniques for 40 days (without missing a day) for the amount of time indicated. Forty days represents a complete mental cycle. The benefits you gain will be yours forever.

As Yogi Bhajan says, "Take meditation to heart as a golden path to infinity which must be experienced in practical activity each day."

The effectiveness of the following techniques will be greatly enhanced if you practice a yoga set, as outlined in this book, before meditating. This will give you some energy to work with, and prime you for the experience.

Maestro,
Your miraculous music heals us,
Restores our sight,
And we shall walk away from anguish,
By your Voice, your Verity,
Your Beauty and Breath,
Your Word and Warmth--
Guiding us to the glad constellation,
Soothing the starved,
Bringing light to lonely hearts--
What opulent ancestry I inherit
When I intone your Name,
When I close my eyes,
I drown in an ocean of Grace.

--Ravi Singh

KIRTAN KRIYA

Kirtan Kriya is one of the most important all-around techniques in Kundalini Yoga. Here's how it's done:

Sit with a straight spine. Your eyes are turned up and in towards the brow. As you chant, whisper, or silently intone the sounds *Sa Ta Na Ma* press the thumbtip of either hand against the corresponding fingertip (figure l).

On *Sa* press the thumb and index fingertips together.
On *Ta* press the thumb and middle fingertips together.
On *Na* press the thumb and ring fingertips together.
On *Ma* press the thumbs and little fingertips together.

Sa Ta Na Ma is chanted in the following melody:

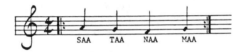

Chant the mantra for 5 minutes. Whisper it for 5 minutes. Do it mentally for 10 minutes, then whisper and chant again for 5 minutes apiece. Feel the sound of the consonants S, T, N, and M, of *Sa Ta Na Ma* coming in through the top of the head, and the "A" sound (as in "MA") going out the brow.

Remember to play the fingers throughout the entire meditation.

To end inhale and stretch your arms straight up. Exhale. Inhale as your twist to the left, exhale center, inhale twist to the right, exhale center. Inhale and stretch up one more time, shake your hands. Sit in silence for a minute before resuming normal activity. The entire time for the meditation is 31 minutes.

Kirtan means Celestial Song. This meditation will allow the Divine melody of Creation to flow through you, heal emotional scars, and help you access and coordinate your total mental and intuitive capacity. Kirtan Kriya also activates the "golden cord," which is considered to be the etheric connection between the pituitary and pineal glands. When this link is established one is able to know the Unknown and see the Unseen.

Kirtan Kriya is very powerful for women in its ability to clear the psyche of the effects of any negative relationship or encounter.

Sa Ta Na Ma means Existence, Life, Death, & Rebirth. The whole mantra means I am the Manifestation of Truth. The fingers relate to specific areas of the brain and aspect of your conscious self.

> *The index or Jupiter finger relates for Wisdom and Knowledge.*
> *The middle or Saturn finger relates to Focus and Discipline.*
> *The ring or Sun finger relates to energy of life and relationship.*
> *The little or Mercury finger relates to communication.*
> *The thumb seals all these attributes into your consciousness.*

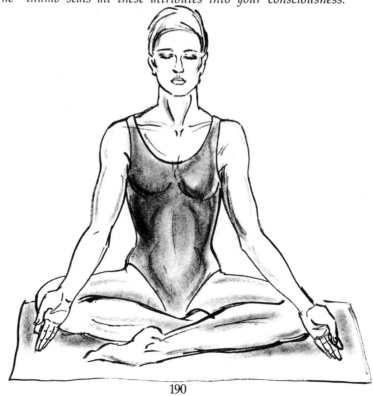

190

LONG SAT NAMS

Have your hands in Prayer Pose (figure 3). Inhale deep and chant a long *SAAAAAAAAT* (the long *Sat* is chanted to almost the full extent of your breath capacity) and a very brief *Nam*. As you do this you can feel *Sat* rising up the spine and *Nam* going out the top of the head. Time open.

Although seemingly simple, this meditation can help you re-establish your equilibrium and give you an overview so that your problems won't weigh heavy on you. You can do this with your family or friends a few times before a meal. Do this with your children to give them a sense of the sacred. Your plants will like it too! In short, long Sat Nams will raise your consciousness.

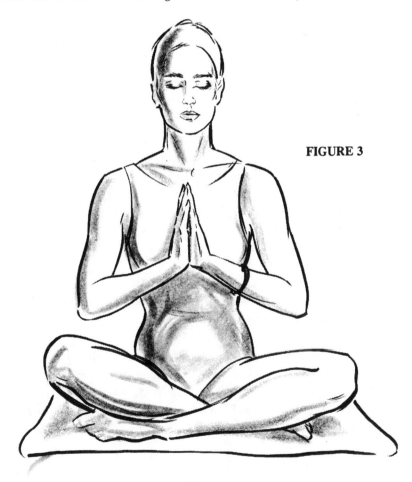

FIGURE 3

MEDITATION TO SEND HEALING ENERGY & HELP HEAL YOURSELF

Sit straight. Your eyes are 1/10 open looking down towards the tip of the nose. Your elbows are bent and pressed down along the sides. Your hands are bent at the wrists and the palms are facing up. Your fingers are angling out to the sides at 45 degrees (figure 4). Keep this angle throughout the entire meditation. There will be a definite pressure on the wrists.

Inhale, then chant *Ra Ma Da Sa* (pause) *Sa Say So Hung* in the following melody:

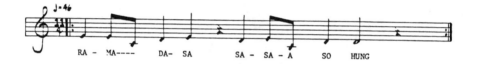

It's chanted in an 11 beat cycle: *Ra Ma Da Sa* (clip this syllable and pause one beat) *Sa Say Sa Hung*. Each syllable is one beat. The last two beats are the inhale, in preparation for the next round. Continue for 11 minutes, then inhale, hold the breath and send love and light to someone you care about. Visualize them as healthy, happy, and fulfilled. Do this visualization twice more.

Ra Ma Da Sa Sa Say So Hung means Sun Moon Earth Infinity, I am that Infinity I belong to and contain. This is a powerful healing mantra. Always use it with reverence and respect.

Remember, Cause and Effect is an inviolable law of the Universe. Whenever we pray or send positive thoughts to someone it has to make a difference. This meditation helps you to channelize and magnify the power of your thoughts, to bring about health and happiness. Whenever we make sacrifices to uplift and heal others, the Universe will sacrifice for us.

FIGURE 4

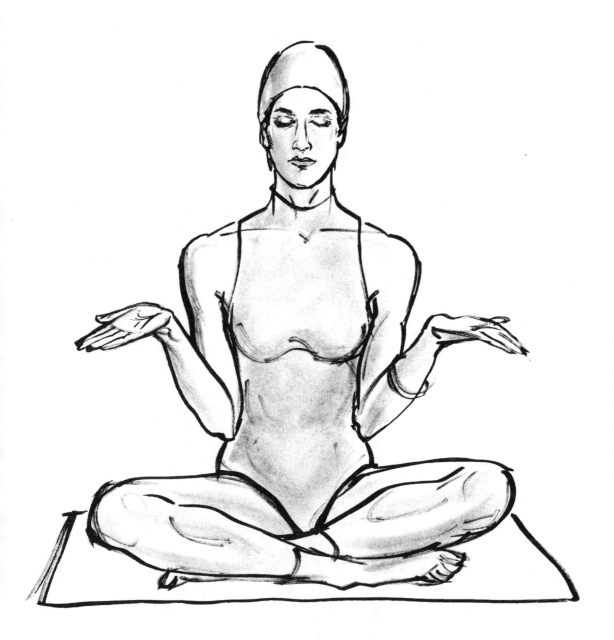

MEDITATION FOR SELF THERAPY

A. Come onto your hands and knees in Cow Pose (figure 7). Press your head up as high as you can, so that your eyes are looking straight up. Breathe long and deeply. After the first minute start thinking of things that bother you. Don't think you have to be "spiritual." If we can let ourselves be ungraceful in this controlled context, then we'll have the ability to be graceful in our lives. Try to think negative and nasty thoughts while breathing in Cow Pose. Breathe out all your pent-up frustrations.

Hold Cow Pose with Long Deep Breathing for 7 minutes.

B. Sit on your heels and lower your forehead to the ground. This is Baby Pose (figure 8). Remember, "Where you bow you will be blessed." Feel protected and perfected, secure, and pure. Remain in Baby Pose for 3-5 minutes.

C. Sit up on your heels, drop your head back. Look up at the sky and laugh! and keep laughing. Time open. (figure 9).

Some people go to various therapists and talk for years, and never seem to get closer to a resolution of what's bothering them. This meditation can help you get to the heart of the matter and work out your frustrations and hidden agendas, so that they don't fester in you and cause you to self-destruct or act in a way you're sorry for later

FIGURE 7

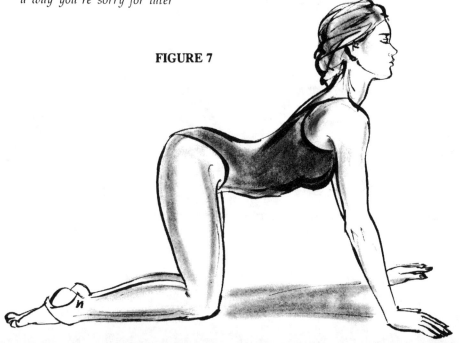

FIGURE 8

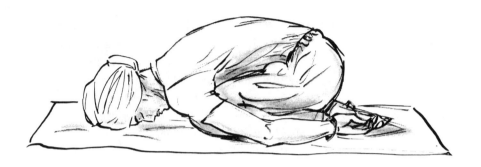

FIGURE 9

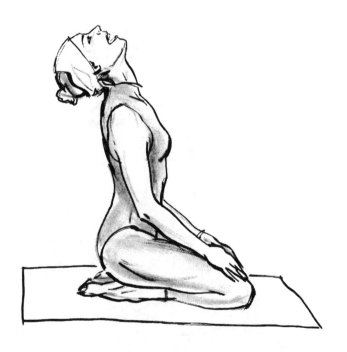

DEEP MEDITATION INTO THOUGHTLESSNESS

Sit with a straight spine and turn your eyes to the brow. Your hands are in your lap, one in the other with both palms up (figure 2). Mentally intone the sound *Wha Hay Gu Ru* in four separate syllables. Hear the sound above the top of the head. Allow yourself to transcend all thoughts, concepts, and expectations. Simply be. Continue for 31 minutes, taking the last minute to stretch Don't rush into anything afterwards. You're higher than you think!

Deep Meditation into Thoughtlessness will help you experience a pure state of being, beyond your thoughts and their polar pull. Did you ever notice that sometimes it's hard to be alone in a room without the television or radio on? We can extend this example to our inner lives We feel lost without our memories, fantasies, and constant mental dialogue. This technique can help you to perceive in fresh and direct ways. It's been said that for most people, the process of thinking is nothing more than a rearranging of prejudices. This meditation can make your mind a mirror and adventures in consciousness something more than someone else's travelogue.

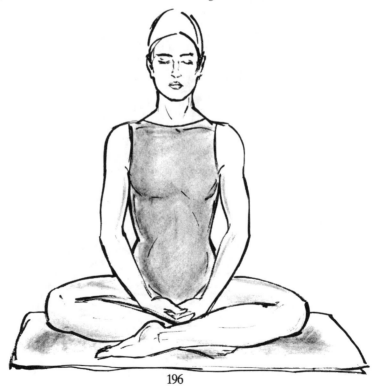

MEDITATION TO COMMUNICATE WITH YOUR SOUL

Sit comfortably with a straight spine. Focus at the brow with the eyes closed (figure 5). Inhale, then chant in a monotone:

Wahay Guru Wahay Guru Wahay Guru Wahay Jio

Do this 8 times per breath. If you can't do it 8 times without having to inhale, then inhale when necessary and build up to 8 repetitions over time. The key to this is to let your diaphragm stay relaxed. Don't force the inhale. You'll be able to take in more breath if you let the inhale be relaxed. It may prove to be somewhat of a tongue twister in the beginning. Persevere!

Stretch upon completion and take your time resuming normal activity.

Wahay Guru means Indescribable Wisdom or Ecstasy beyond words. Jio means O my soul. The entire mantra means O my soul, God is. This meditation brings balance to your being, and eliminates negativity. Do it for 31 minutes.

This mantra is unique in its ability to not only balance your brain areas, but integrate their activity as well.

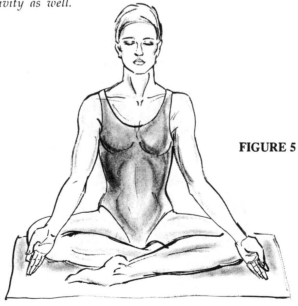

FIGURE 5

SLOW BREATH WITH SAT NAM WAHAY GURU

Sit with a straight spine, focus at the brow (figure 5). As you inhale slowly, mentally intone *Sat Nam* 16 times in a gently pulsating rhythm. As you exhale mentally intone *Wahay Guru* 16 times in a gently pulsating rhythm.

The ideal is to have both the inhale and exhale take 20-30 seconds (or more) each, so you're in effect breathing 1 time per minute. The breath is silk thread, long and smooth.

Do this for 11 minutes initially, and build up to 31 minutes over time.

Long Slow Breathing helps you master your mind and environments. In addition, it allows your body's self-healing mechanisms to activate.

The claims for this meditation are that it engenders a powerful state of health and vibrancy, and brings exalted consciousness. It's said that mastery of this technique will help you increase your capacity to heal others through touch.

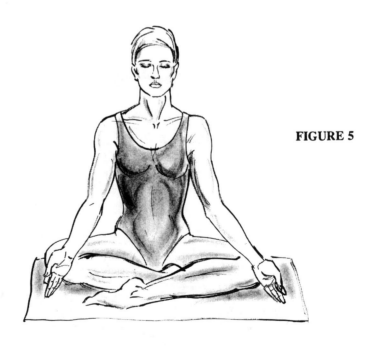

FIGURE 5

MEDITATION FOR INSIGHT AND THE POWER OF THE WORD

Sit with a straight spine. The hands are in *gyan mudra*. The thumb and index finger tips are meeting. Press the back of the tongue against the roof of the mouth. Your teeth are pressed together, front teeth to front teeth, molar to molar. Apply Neck Lock. Your eyes are 1/10 open, looking down towards the tip of the nose (figure 5).

Mentally intone the sounds *Sa Ta Na Ma*. Project out the brow, as you focus at the tip of the nose. In a sense, your awareness is in two places at once. At the brow, and the tip of the nose.

Ideally, you should practice this for at least 31 minutes, and if possible longer. If you apply yourself diligently, it's possible to master this meditation in one sitting, and accrue many inner benefits which will be yours for a lifetime.

This meditation will give you powerful intuition, and a knowledge of the outcome of your intended actions. It will also give your words a penetrating quality. In fact, this meditation gives gifts to almost everyone who practices it sincerely. It's been my experience that this meditation engenders eloquence, and is very effective when I'm feeling mentally stressed or over-extended.

This technique will give your glandular system a tune-up. It's very powerful when practiced on the eve of a full moon.

RAJA YOGA MEDITATION

Sit with a straight spine. Be aware of the flow of the breath. Feel it as a life giving current. Be aware of which nostril is more open. Long Deep Breathing 3 minutes.

Bring your awareness to the First Center of Consciousness at the rectum. Inhale and squeeze the rectum muscle. Exhale and release it. Continue for 1 minute.

Now be aware of the sex organ. As you inhale squeeze the rectum and sex organ. As you exhale release these muscles. Continue for 1 minute.

Concentrate on your navel. As you inhale pull the rectum sex organ, and navel. Feel the energy mixing at the navel. Exhale. Continue for 1 minute.

Concentrate at the Heart Center, which lies in the area of the sternum. Contract the rectum, sex organ, and navel point. In addition pull the diaphragm up under the ribs. Maintaining these locks, breathe long and deeply. Breathe from the base of the spine to the Heart Center area.

Now continue to breathe and apply *Maha Bhand*. Contract the rectum, sex organ, navel, diaphragm, and apply neck lock. The chin is pulled back so that the neck is straight. Turn your eyes up towards the top of the head. Visualize the spine as a glowing rod. Continue for 3 minutes. Then inhale, exhale. hold the breath out. Inhale and relax the breath.

Again apply all the locks. Inhale, hold the breath and pump your belly 5 times. Exhale. Inhale, hold the breath and pump your belly 8 times. Continue this pattern and pump your belly 10, 12, 17, 22, 24, and 26 times with the breath held.

Now do Long Deep Breathing. Move the energy along the spine to the pineal gland in the center of the brain. Continue with focus for up to 11 minutes.

Hold your knees. Press your lower spine forward. Focus your eyes at the brow. Breath of Fire for 3 minutes.

Now chant the sound *Hum*, letting the "m" sound resonate at the sternum. Continue at a pace slightly faster than one time per second for 3 minutes. *Hum* means "we." It's a Heart Center sound.

Turn your eyes to the top of the head. Chant a long *Ong*. The sound is very nasal, so that it vibrates your skull bones. Merge with the Cosmos. Feel all of Creation chanting with you. 3 minutes.

Meditate and listen as the Universe continues to chant.

Raja Yoga entails mental concentration and visualization for the systematic raising of consciousness towards Union with the Divine.

This meditation will give you a working knowledge of the chakras (see appendix 11). You will be moving your awareness through the important energy centers along the spine.

You will also gain insight into the connection between the mind and the breath, and arrive at an experience of higher consciousness.

As you proceed through this sequence don't force the breath. Be systematic, and increase the time over time.

MEDITATION TO BE CAPABLE AND CALM

Sit comfortably. Have your left wrist on the left knee, palm facing up. With the four fingers of the right hand, find the pulse on the upturned left wrist. The pulse is usually felt on the thumb side of the tendon that runs up the center of the forearm. Close your eyes and focus up at the brow. With every pulse mentally intone *Sat Nam*. Let the sound toll you deeper and deeper into your self (figure 6). 11 minutes.

Let your mind be quiescent
No more to roam,
Find that place of inner peace,
Your true ancestral home.

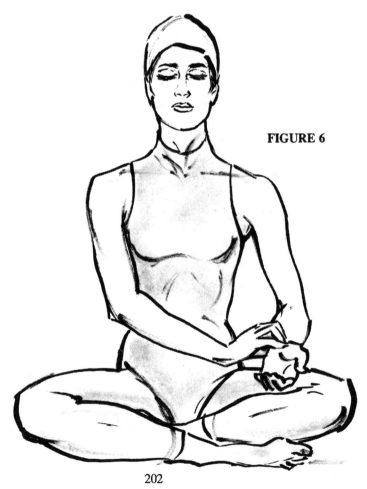

FIGURE 6

How can I assay your worth
When gold is destitute next to you--
Most rare jewel of all my days.
Make me a spoke in the wheel of those
Who are forever turning in praise.

--Ravi Singh

What was I in lieu of You--
Delinquent in my love for You.
It's part of the story
In which I wanted to come to You
But never would.
Now my soul's tattooed with your Name.

O my One,
It's with the mind You gave us that we forget you,
And by your Grace
That our Love for You out of longing is born.

--Ravi Singh

Appendix 1 - The Chakras

The *chakras* are fountains of energy which lie along the spine. Each *chakra* represents an aspect of consciousness, mode of behavior, perspective, and is an etheric counterpart to an important nerve center or gland.

Your understanding of this model will enable you to assess where you are on the path of self-growth, and help others accordingly.

The *chakras* are rungs on the ladder of light, which rise from the mundane to the miraculous, from a fate to a Destiny.

There are eight major *chakras*. When our energy is flowing freely through all of them, we can easily be complete and fulfilled.

The First *Chakra* is at the rectum. Its frequency corresponds to the color red, and its quality to the element earth. This center relates to elimination, instinct, survival, habits, and represents the realm of the quotidian, ordinary day to day life.

When our energy is flowing freely through the First Center we are grounded, dependable, realistic, and secure.

If energy is stuck here there's a tendency to be clinging, coarse, overly stubborn, and exhibit signs of an addictive or anal retentive personality. First Center imbalances also manifest as very ungrounded or spacey behavior.

The First Center holds subconscious patterns. Deep insecurities, and neurotic or perverse behavior are examples of First Center imbalances.

The Second *Chakra* is a nerve center that relates to the sex organ. Its frequency corresponds to the color orange, and its quality is that of water. It is the realm of sensation.

When energy is flowing freely through this center a person is expressive, balanced in relationship, and has a personal flare, and a sense of individuality.

If energy is stuck at the Second Center one tends to be overly-obsessed with sex and its cultural accoutrements, or overly puritanical in relation to it.

The Third Center corresponds to the Navel Point/Solar Plexus area. Its frequency corresponds to saffron-yellow, and its quality is that of fire. It is the seat of power, and is a reservoir for the energy of life.

When energy is flowing freely through this center a person is focused and fearless. They have a strong will and are successful in life.

When the energy is blocked here, a person tends to exploit others or is too easily exploited. There is also a tendency to be drunk on emotions, intensity, passion or power.

The first three centers or Lower Triangle, relate to the mind, its patterns and persuasions. The higher centers, relate to the spirit and higher potential. ideally the lower centers give us a base or framework for the expression of the higher.

The 4th center is called the Heart Center. It lies in the area of the sternum. Its frequency corresponds to the color green and its quality to the element air. It relates to love, expansion, and the indefatigable nature of the human spirit.

When the Heart Center is open you begin to get a sense of your Infinite identity. You have the capacity to sacrifice for the sake of sacrifice, and love unqualifiedly. The Heart Center is the first center of higher consciousness.

An imbalance at the Heart Center often renders a person incapable of saying no, in other words they overextend themselves, or feel overwhelmed by their feelings It may also result in hardheartedness, lack of compassion, and manic behavior.

The Fifth Center is the throat center, which relates to the thyroid gland. Its frequency corresponds to the color light blue and its quality to the element ether. Through the Throat Center we give substance to idea. It is the seat of creativity.

When energy is flowing through the Throat Center we have the ability to command, and speak eloquently, and are able to translate our concepts into reality, speak the truth and live the truth. When the Throat Center is blocked we feel creatively stifled, and have difficulty being direct and truthful in our dealings with others.

The Sixth Center is called the Third Eye or *Ajna Chakra*. Its frequency relates to the color indigo. Its quality is beyond quality. Through the Sixth Center we master our minds and pierce the veil of illusion. Our awareness here is focus itself. The Third Eye corresponds to the pituitary gland. When the Third Eye is in balance, we have a meditative mind, the ability to know the Unknown, see the Unseen and an an understanding of our Destiny.

The 7th Center, at the top of the head, is called the Thousand Petalled Lotus, or the seat of the soul. Its relative frequency corresponds to the color violet. It relates to the pineal gland. When the 7th Center is in balance we feel part of the vastness of all that is. The experience here is ecstasy beyond words.

The 8th Center is your aura, and represents the working balance of all the centers, our ability to integrate higher conscious into our presence and projection.

APPENDIX 2 - THE TEN BODIES

The model of the ten bodies is an archetype which describes aspects of our totality in a multi-dimensional sense. When the ten bodies are all formed, and working in unison, they merge into the 11th body which represents the perfected being.

The First Body of Light is the Soul Body. It represents our very essence, uncomplicated and pure. It's that quiet but insistent inner voice which inspires us towards God.

When we refuse to recognize the promptings of our soul, we find ourselves embroiled in conflicts between our head and heart. Sometimes we have to circumvent "reason" to give sustenance to our soul.

The Second Body of Light is called the Negative Mind, and it helps us to calculate possible pitfalls in any given situation. People whose negative minds are not in balance, frequently find themselves giving away their power, out of a tremendous need to connect with others in various kinds of relationships.

To master our second body we must be able to transform emotion into devotion. In other words we have to choose to "fall in love" with the things which will never let us down i.e. yoga, a True Teacher who inspires us to Infinity, a path with heart, and God and His Grand Design.

The Third Body of Light is called the Positive Mind and it relates to our optimistic side, the ability to give hope to all. When our Positive Minds are imbalanced we tend to be negative and depressed, void of hope.

The Fourth Body of Light is called the Neutral Mind. The Neutral Mind is not a given but has to be developed through meditation. It represents the ability to see both sides of every issue and arrive at the course of action or insight which is in our overall best interest.

The neutral or non-discriminating mind is one of the highest attainments in yoga, it leads to Liberation.

The Fifth Body of Light is the Physical Body. In the ultimate sense a person who masters this aspect is able to sacrifice their comfort, well-being, safety, and even their life, to lead others to an experience of Infinity. This is the domain of a True Teacher, who puts his/her body on the line to be Divine.

When a person's Fifth Body is not integrated they tend to be very indulgent and lazy. The remedy is to move. Exercise, dance, walk, run, and above all to Kundalini Yoga!

This Sixth Body of Light is called the Arcline. It relates to the beaming power of the mind, the ability to project to Infinity and get a corresponding readout in reality. This is the power of prayer.

When The Arcline is strong a person is intuitive, focused, and successful. When one's Arcline is weak, a person can be scattered and accident prone.

The Seventh Body of Light is your Aura or Magnetic Field. When this is strong you have the ability to heal, uplift, and inspire by your very presence. You have charisma.

When your Magnetic Field is weak you tend to repel rather than attract people, and frequently feel overlooked and anonymous. People with weak auras have a greater tendency to be in the wrong place at the wrong time.

Ultimately all true and enduing communication takes place on an auric level, that is as an interchange between Magnetic Fields. Ponder this deeply!

The Eighth Body of Light is called the *Pranic* Body, and relates to energy and fearlessness. When it's strong you have the ability to regenerate very effectively and keep going. All forms of yogic breathing which we practice in Kundalini Yoga activate the *Pranic* Body. Remember when you master your breathing you master your mind.

The Pranic Body feeds in through the adrenals. When the *Pranic* Body is strong you have the ability to get "jazzed up," and impart energy to all those around you.

The Ninth Body of Light is called the Subtle Body and it relates to Mastery, the ability to know the Unknown and see the Unseen, to read between the lines, and see beneath the surface.

When your ninth body is not integrated you tend to be very insensitive, awkward, and somewhat scattered. To develop the subtle body we must learn to be sensitive to our sensitivity. Yogis tell us that the Subtle Body is the capsule which conveys the soul to its Destination at the time of Death.

The Tenth Body of Light is called the Radiant Body. It relates to nerve strength, royal courage, and the ability to stand out and take a stand. It's your warrior aspect, all or nothing.

The Eleventh Body of Light, as stated, is the crystallization of the ten bodies. To accomplish this, one must transcend one's narrowness, deliver and dedicate oneself to a path with heart, and bow to its Teachings.

209

APPENDIX 3 - KUNDALINI YOGA MANTRAS

Many of the mantras which follow were not presented in this book but play an important role in many Kundalini Yoga techniques. If you continue your practice through our Teaching Centers, or obtain some of the addition books and tapes we offer, you'll no doubt encounter some of these.

Ad Guray Namay, Jugad Guray Namay, Sat Guray Namay, Siri Guru Dev A Namay - I Bow to the Primal Wisdom, I Bow to the Wisdom Through the Ages, I Bow to the True Wisdom, I Bow to the Great Unseen Wisdom.

Ap Sahaee Hoa Suchay Da Such A Doa - I Take Refuge in the True One; The True One is My True Support, God, God, God.

Ardas Bayee, Amar Das Guru, Amar Das Guru Ardas Bayee, Ram Das Guru, Ram Das Guru, Ram Das Guru, Suchee Sahee - The Fulfillment of Your Prayers is Guaranteed by the Grace of Guru Amar Das (The Hope for the Hopeless) and Guru Ram Das (King of the Yogis and Bestower of Blessings), Past, Present, and Future, Signed, Sealed. and Delivered.

Ek Ong Kar, Sat Nam, Siri Wahe Guru - There is One Creator Who is Your True Identity. There are No Words for that Wisdom Which is Ecstasy.

Ek Ong Kar, Sat Nam, Karta Purkh, Nir Bhau, Nir Vair, Akal Mort, Ajuni, Say Bhang, Gurprasad, Jap, Ad Such, Jugad Such, Habee Such, Nanaka Hosee Be Such - There's One Creator, The Doer of Everything, Fearless, Revengeless, Unborn, Undying. and Self-Illumined, This is Revealed Through the True Guru's Grace. Meditate!, True in the Beginning, True Through All Time, True Now, O Nanak the True One Shall Ever be True.

Gobinday, Mukunday, Udaray, Uparay, Hariang, Kariang, Near-Nomay, Akamay - Sustainer, Liberator, Enlightener, Infinite, Destroyer, Creator, Nameless, Desireless.

Guru Guru Wahay Guru, Guru Ram Das Guru - The Wisdom Which Comes as a Servant of the Infinite.

Har - The Creative Aspect of Infinity

210

Ong Namo Guru Dev Namo - Infinite Creative Consciousness I Call on You, Divine Wisdom Within I Call on You.
Ra Ma Da Sa Sa Say So Hung - Sun, Moon, Earth, Infinity, I am that Infinity I belong to and contain.

Sat Nam - True Identity

Sa Ta Na Ma - Existence, Life, Death, Rebirth

Sat Narien, Wahay Guru, Hari Narien, Sat Nam - Clear Perception of Truth, Ecstasy Beyond Words, Clear Perception of the Creative Essence of the Divine, Truth is God's Name.

Wahay Guru, Wahay Guru, Wahay Guru, Wahay Jio - O my Soul God is.

Wahay Guru - Ecstasy Beyond Words

Wha Yantay, Kar Yantay, Juga Duta Patee, Adaka It Whaha, Brahmaday, Taysha Guru, It a Wahay Guru - Great Macroself, Creative Self, All That is Creative Through Time, All That is the Great One, 3 Aspects of God (Generating, Organizing, Destroying) are contained in Wahay Guru.

Many of the *mantras* presented in this book, along with other inspiring offerings, can be enjoyed on tape with musical accomppaniment. For more information call Invincible Recordings at 1-800-275-2022 or White Lion Press at 1-800-243-9642.

APPENDIX 4 - KUNDALINI YOGA TEACHING CENTERS

No matter where you live on planet earth, chances are that Kundalini Yoga classes are given somewhere near. For more information please contact either of the following:

3HO-Foundation
International Headquarters
PO Box 351149
Los Angeles,California 90035
(213)552-3416

Ravi Singh Kundalini Yoga
c/o White Lion Press
225 E. 5th St. #4D
New York, NY 10003
(212)475-0212

ABOUT THE AUTHOR

Ravi Singh is putting Kundalini Yoga on the map! For the past 20 years, in New York City, and nationwide, he's been gaining wide recognition as a dynamic and inspiring Teacher. Mr. Singh has taught in many contexts. He's worked with Olympic Athletes, Scientists at Bell Laboratories, Opera Singers at the Aspen Music Festival, Executives at major corporations, and many Artists in the creative and performing arts, including such notables as Liv Ullman, and Yehudi Menuhan, and dancers from the Martha Graham, Merce Cunningham, Trisha Brown, David Gordon, & Jose Limon dance companies.

As Director for the New York Center for Art & Awareness, Mr. Singh offers classes which bring the ancient technology of Yoga into a modern framework.

Mr. Singh's approach is both powerful and poetic, meditative and moving. As an accomplished poet his books include: *Small Poems to God*, & *Long Song to the One I Love*..

Ravi Singh has the following Books and Videos Available:

Books:

Kundalini Yoga for Strength, Success, & Spirit - $15.95

Videotapes:

Kundalini Yoga w/Ravi Singh -	$28.95
Ultimate Stretch/Warrior Workout -	$29.95
The Kundalini Experience -	$29.95
Long Live You! -	$28.95
Navel Power -	$28.95
Golden Yoga (for Seniors) -	$28.95

For Information on Ravi Singh's classes, to order the book and tapes listed above (Visa/MC accepted) call 1-800-243-9642 or write:

White Lion Press
225 E. 5th St. #4D
New York, New York 10003